DATE DUE

U. C. FEB 13 '82 APR 29 '85			
GAYLORD			PRINTED IN U.S.A.

REHABILITATION TECHNIQUES IN SEVERE DISABILITY

Publication Number 926
AMERICAN LECTURE SERIES®

A Publication in
The BANNERSTONE DIVISION *of*
AMERICAN LECTURES IN SOCIAL AND REHABILITATION PSYCHOLOGY

Editors of the Series

RICHARD E. HARDY, Ed.D.

Chairman, Department of
Rehabilitation Counseling
Virginia Commonwealth University
Richmond, Virginia

and

JOHN G. CULL, Ph.D.

Director, Regional Counselor Training Program
Department of Rehabilitation Counseling
Virginia Commonwealth University
Fishersville, Virginia

The American Lecture Series in Social and Rehabilitation Psychology offers books which are concerned with man's role in his milieu. Emphasis is placed on how this role can be made more effective in a time of social conflict and a deteriorating physical environment. The books are oriented toward descriptions of what future roles should be and are not concerned exclusively with the delineation and definition of contemporary behavior. Contributors are concerned to a considerable extent with prediction through the use of a functional view of man as opposed to a descriptive anatomical point of view.

Books in this series are written mainly for the professional practitioner; however, academicians will find them of considerable value in both undergraduate and graduate courses in the helping services.

Rehabilitation Techniques In Severe Disability

CASE STUDIES

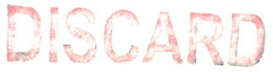

JOHN G. CULL

RICHARD E. HARDY

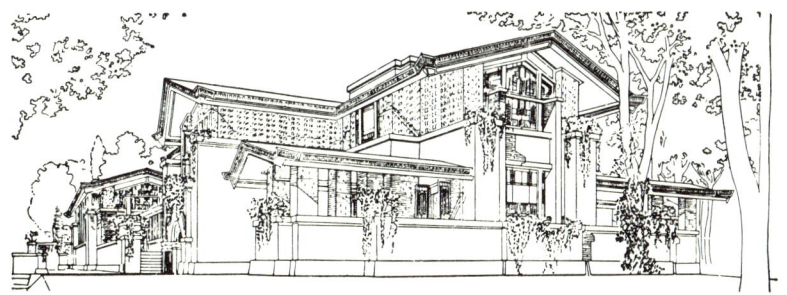

Andrew S. Thomas Memorial Library
MORRIS HARVEY COLLEGE, CHARLESTON, W. VA.

CHARLES C THOMAS • PUBLISHER
Springfield · Illinois · U.S.A.

362
C897re

Published and Distributed Throughout the World by
CHARLES C THOMAS • PUBLISHER
Bannerstone House
301-327 East Lawrence Avenue, Springfield, Illinois, U.S.A.

This book is protected by copyright. No part of it may be reproduced in any manner without written permission from the publisher.

©*1974, by* CHARLES C THOMAS • PUBLISHER
ISBN 0-398-02963-6
Library of Congress Catalog Card Number: 73-11437

With THOMAS BOOKS *careful attention is given to all details of manufacturing and design. It is the Publisher's desire to present books that are satisfactory as to their physical qualities and artistic possibilities and appropriate for their particular use.* THOMAS BOOKS *will be true to those laws of quality that assure a good name and good will.*

Printed in the United States of America
R-1

Library of Congress Cataloging in Publication Data
Cull, John G.
 Rehabilitation techniques in severe disability.
 (American lecture series, publication no. 926. A publication in the Bannerstone division of American lectures in social and rehabilitation psychology)
 1. Rehabilitation—United States—Case studies—Addresses, essays, lectures. 2. Rehabilitation counseling—Case studies—Addresses, essays, lectures. I. Hardy, Richard E., joint author. II. Title.
 [DNLM: 1. Handicapped—Collected works. 2. Rehabilitation—Collected works. HD7256.U5 C967r 1974]
 HD7256.U5Cg37   362.1   73-11437
 ISBN 0-398-02963-6

CONTRIBUTORS

ROY W. BROOKS, Chief of Physical Restoration Services, Division of Vocational Rehabilitation, Illinois State Board of Vocational Education and Rehabilitation.

JOHN G. CULL, Ph.D., Director, Regional Counselor Training Program and Professor, Department of Rehabilitation Counseling, School of Community Services, Virginia Commonwealth University.

R. WILLIAM ENGLISH, Assistant Professor and Coordinator of Clinical Activities of the Rehabilitation Counselor Education Program, Syracuse University.

ARNOLD H. FREEDMAN, Senior Rehabilitation Counselor, Division of Vocational Rehabilitation, Connecticut State Board of Education.

A. G. GARRIS, Rehabilitation Consultant, California State Department of Rehabilitation.

ANN GLASS, Rehabilitation Counselor, California State Department of Rehabilitation.

RICHARD E. HARDY, Ed.D., Chairman and Professor, Department of Rehabilitation Counseling. School of Community Services, Virginia Commonwealth University.

PARNELL McLAUGHLIN, Ed.D., Director, Division of Rehabilitation, Colorado State Department of Social Services.

SEYMOUR MUND, Senior Rehabilitation Counselor, Division of Vocational Rehabilitation, Connecticut State Board of Education.

AUBREY E. NEELEY, Supervisor of Rehabilitation Services, Division of Rehabilitation and Crippled Children, Alabama State Department of Education.

CLINTON S. VIETH, Assistant Director, South Dakota Service to the Visually Impaired.

JOHN H. WEBB, A.E.S., Director, Division of Vocational Rehabilitation, Mississippi State Department of Education.

This book is dedicated to

Otho Howard Smith

of Virginia

For outstanding leadership in services to handicapped persons

PREFACE

THE contributors to this book were carefully selected from throughout the United States. Only those persons with considerable experience in rehabilitation services and who could articulate the special problems of individuals through case study descriptions were asked to be involved in the development of this book.

It should be noted that the material is presented not as all inclusive information but as resource data for discussion groups in introductory rehabilitation classes and orientation sessions of newly employed personnel in rehabilitation programs. The material is, then, meant to provide a "springboard" for extending discussion concerning the effects of disability and rehabilitation services to disabled individuals. This book could also be considered a companion piece to the textbook *Severe Disability: Social and Rehabilitation Approaches* although it is not totally designed for that purpose.

While specific discussion questions and suggested readings are offered after each section, the questions which follow may also be useful to both student and instructor.

1. What are the special problems of this disability group?
    a. medical
    b. psychological
    c. social
    d. vocational
    e. other

What counseling services were provided?
    a. vocational
    b. personal
    c. educational
    d. other

2. What additional services should have been offered or could have been offered?
   a. medical
   b. other psychological
   c. other social
   d. other

3. Was this helpee (client) eligible for vocational rehabilitation services through the state agency? Yes____ No____ On what basis?

   What type of diagnostic information was needed in order to evaluate the vocational plan?

   How was the vocational objective decided in this case?

4. Could this person's problems been dealt with differently — to improve services to him — what would you have done?

5. How were the services of other professionals, including psychologists, physicians, occupational therapists, etc. coordinated by the counselor?

   Did other professional persons understand what the counselor really needed from them in order to help the helpee?

6. Was there documented reporting back to other involved professional team workers?

7. Was the case recorded adequately? Yes____ No____ Why?

8. Was the client involved in all decision making?

9. What were the helpee's real concerns? Did he really get the services he wanted?

10. What were the concerns of the counselor?

11. Were there adequate follow-along services?

12. Are social and rehabilitation services in your state less than adequate, adequate, or more than adequate for this disability group? How? Why?

13. How would the helpee evaluate rehabilitation services?

14. What other questions should be asked in order to evaluate rehabilitation services to the helpee?

The book represents an enormous amount of work on the part of the contributors and the editors in that it was necessary to carefully select those descriptions which should be presented in order to give the reader the information he needs to increase his understanding of these special problems. Many descriptions were written only to be discarded and the effort begun again. We owe a real debt of gratitude to those who worked so hard with us on this project and call your special attention to their names and institutional affiliations. We are especially indebted to Dr. English for his fine "lead off" chapter.

JOHN G. CULL
RICHARD E. HARDY

CONTENTS

	Page
Contributors	v
Preface	ix

Chapter

1. The Application of Personality Theory to Explain Reactions to Physical Disability ... 3
2. The Epileptic ... 21
3. Case Study — Spinal Cord Injury ... 33
4. Case Study of Pulmonary Condition ... 48
5. Case Study of Cardiovascular Disease ... 62
6. Mental Retardation ... 75
7. The Visually Impaired ... 88
8. The Diabetic ... 99
9. The Blind Diabetic ... 104
10. Cancer ... 122
11. Deafness and Its Effects ... 138
12. The Amputee ... 158
13. Rheumatoid Arthritis ... 184
14. The Drug Abuser ... 200

Appendix ... 229
Index ... 231

REHABILITATION TECHNIQUES IN SEVERE DISABILITY

The following books have appeared thus far in the Social and Rehabilitation Psychology Series:

A BOOK OF READINGS IN MENTAL RETARDATION AND PHYSICAL DISABILITY
Richard E. Hardy and John G. Cull

UNDERSTANDING DISABILITY FOR SOCIAL AND REHABILITATION SERVICES
John G. Cull and Richard E. Hardy

REHABILITATION OF THE URBAN DISADVANTAGED
John G. Cull and Richard E. Hardy

THE NEGLECTED OLDER AMERICAN – SOCIAL AND REHABILITATION SERVICES
John G. Cull and Richard E. Hardy

FUNDAMENTALS OF CRIMINAL BEHAVIOR AND CORRECTIONAL SYSTEMS
John G. Cull and Richard E. Hardy

THE BIG WELFARE MESS – PUBLIC ASSISTANCE AND REHABILITATION APPROACHES
John G. Cull and Richard E. Hardy

ADJUSTMENT TO WORK
John G. Cull and Richard E. Hardy

VOCATIONAL EVALUATION FOR REHABILITATION SERVICES
Richard E. Hardy and John G. Cull

REHABILITATION OF THE DRUG ABUSER WITH DELINQUENT BEHAVIOR
Richard E. Hardy and John G. Cull

INTRODUCTION TO CORRECTIONAL REHABILITATION
Richard E. Hardy and John G. Cull

DRUG DEPENDENCE AND REHABILITATION APPROACHES
Richard E. Hardy and John G. Cull

CLIMBING GHETTO WALLS
Richard E. Hardy and John G. Cull

CONTEMPORARY FIELD WORK PRACTICES IN REHABILITATION
John G. Cull and Craig R. Colvin

VOCATIONAL REHABILITATION: PROFESSION AND PROCESS
John G. Cull and Richard E. Hardy

MEDICAL AND PSYCHOLOGICAL ASPECTS OF DISABILITY
A. Beatrix Cobb

SPECIAL PROBLEMS IN REHABILITATION
A. Beatrix Cobb

SEVERE DISABILITIES: SOCIAL AND REHABILITATION APPROACHES
Richard E. Hardy and John G. Cull

Chapter 1

THE APPLICATION OF PERSONALITY THEORY TO EXPLAIN PSYCHOLOGICAL REACTIONS TO PHYSICAL DISABILITY

R. WILLIAM ENGLISH

Salient Theories in the Psychology of Disability
Overview
Concluding Remarks
Discussion Questions
References and Suggested Reading

IN spite of a considerable increase, in recent years, in efforts to research many areas of rehabilitation psychology, virtually nothing has been done to relate salient personality theories to a developing psychology of disability. Although a little is known as to "why" physically disabled persons react as they do to disablement (McDaniel, 1969), even less is known about "why" the physically disabled are stigmatized (Yuker, Block and Campbell, 1966, and English, 1971).

In this sense, the chapter that follows is something of a pioneering effort where precedents are lacking. Because this is a theoretical study, the goal will be to develop a manuscript that is basically descriptive and hypothesis-generating.

SALIENT THEORIES IN THE PSYCHOLOGY OF DISABILITY

Certain major theoretical principles and positions have obtained popularity in the psychology of chronic illness and disability and have more potential value than others. Occasionally these theories have been used to try and explain the impact of disablement on disabled persons *per se;* however, it seems possible to apply the same constructs to explain stigma.) The theories that will be examined are: (1) Psychoanalytic Theory; (2) Individual Psychology; (3) Body Image Theory; and (4) Social Role Theory.

Psychoanalytic Theory

The earliest theory of personality which has applicability to explaining a psychology of disability is that of psychoanalytic theory developed by Sigmund Freud in the late 1800's and early 1900's. Freud conceptualized a duality of existence, where people are humans and animals. Within this model, he believed that people exist at different levels of growth and development, the lowest levels corresponding to the basic animal side of man. At lower maturational levels, psychoanalytic theory suggests that man operates in accordance with basic instinctual drives involving sex and security needs where only the fittest individuals survive. A central tenet of psychoanalytic theory seems to be that "competition" rules the lives of men. Where there is little if any security, the struggle between men may be very physical, resulting in the death or injury of combatants. However, even when physical security is virtually assured, as has generally been the case since the industrial revolution, men continue to compete for "psychological superiority." Psychoanalytic theorists believe that most behavior is unconscious and that learned behavior occurs in the formative preschool years.

If this bird's eye view of psychoanalytic theory is applied to stigma, we might hypothesize that a nondisabled person who is prejudiced towards the disabled is a relatively immature individual with unexpressed hostilities and a need to feel psychologically superior. In terms of the disabled themselves, psychoanalytic theories would believe that disablement almost always has an adverse effect on personality, especially if it occurs in early childhood. They are likely to be immature and passive-aggressive types. Persons disabled after school begins probably would not experience any substantial change in personality, according to psychoanalytic thinking.

Individual Psychology

A neo-psychoanalytic theory of personality which is often mentioned by students of disability is termed "individual psychology." Its author was Alfred Adler (1927), who studied psychiatry with Freud after practicing ophthalmology and general medicine in Vienna. Adler's personality theory departed from Freud's psychoanalytic theory in its emphasis on social motivation and individuality, rather than sexual impulses.

The most relevant of Adler's constructs that relate to the stigmatization of the physically disabled are "striving for superiority," "inferiority," "compensation" and the idea of the "life style." Adler believed that all people possess an innate drive to strive for superiority. He felt this drive evolved into a pattern or life style from early childhood and that it was motivated to compensate for certain innate feelings of inferiority. Stigma, in the view of individual psychology, is part of the life style to achieve superiority, even at others' expense, by nondisabled persons.

Proponents of individual psychology believe that physically disabled persons attempt to compensate for a defective organ by strengthening it. In their view, physical or mental deformities are principal causes of a "faulty" life style. Individual psychology theorists probably believe there is a higher incidence of emotional disturbance among the disabled than the nondisabled (McDaniel, 1969).

Body Image Theory

Another neo-psychoanalytic system prominent in explaining the psychology of disability is "body image theory." The idea of the body image and its disruption due to chronic illness and physical disability has become nearly as popular a construct among rehabilitation practitioners as the construct of "inferiority" (McDaniel, 1969).

The individual who has contributed more than anyone else to body image theory is Paul Schilder (1950), as far back as 1935.

Schilder and others believe that people respond to each other substantially in terms of nonverbal and physical cues and images.

Followers of Gestalt Psychology believe that, over time, most people have come to recognize that there is frequently an inconsistency between verbal and cognitive behavior and nonverbal body behavior (Kohler, 1947). This aspect of our humanness seems recognized both within ourselves and in others. To illustrate, we know there are times we have told companions we are very satisfied while at the exact same moment our gestures and expressions communicated something else. As an aside, it is interesting to note that frequently we are less sensitive to our own incongruence than are others. Based on self-perceptions, it is usually the rule that we place most of our faith in what we see and not what we hear.

Related to this, body image theorists believe that the attitudes individuals have towards themselves and others is viewed as being shaped substantially in terms of their perceptions about physique. Although it is somewhat oversimplified, "body image" can be viewed as a construct existing on a continuum, where those who are most acceptant of their own bodies will be most acceptant of the bodies of others and vice versa.

Theoretically, the construct "body image" is of course closely related to that of the "self-concept," although proponents of Body Image Theory believe they are not equivalent concepts, but rather, that body perceptions reflect generalized feelings of self (Wapner and Warner, 1965). In Freud's early writings he argued that the body image is closely related to the development of the ego. Freud thought the self-core followed first and foremost from a body ego, that the ego is derived from bodily sensations which can be thought of as a mental projection of the surface of the body (Fisher and Cleveland, 1968).

Many body image theorists believe that body attitudes are often the result and reflection of interpersonal relationships. Cleveland (1960) discovered that body attitudes appear to change during psychotherapy, and Popper (1957) showed that body images are differentially affected by previous success and failure experiences. In related research, Cleveland and Fisher (1965) have observed that body feelings are often correlated with various personality measures. Abel (1953) discovered that more severely facially disfigured persons make more distorted figure drawings. Abel's (1953) findings, however, are contradicted by a study by Silverstein and Robinson (1956), who found that judges were unable to distinguish between the self-figure drawings of paralytic and normal children.

Some objective data has come forth with regard to persons objective body image, that is how they are viewed by others, and attitudes towards physically disabled persons. In one study, English and Oberle (1971) had psychiatrists identify the extremes in occupational groups believed to employ women with a high and low emphasis on physique. Using the Attitude Towards Disabled Persons Scale, they found that the high physique group, airline stewardesses, were significantly more rejecting of disabled persons than the low physique group, typists. In another study, Witkin, Lewis, Hertzman, Machover, Meissner and Wapner (1954) demonstrated fairly convincingly that body image is important in determining perceptual functioning. They observed that persons who produced more field dependent figure drawings reflected a lower evaluation or confidence in their own bodies, whereas persons who drew less field dependent figures had more self-body confidence.

Social Role Theory

A relatively recent trend of thought which is valuable to the study of psychological responses to disability and rehabilitation is social role theory. The major contributor in this area has been Talcott Parsons, a sociologist (1951 and 1958).

A basic construct in role theory is that of a "status" which is simply a collection of rights and duties (Linton, 1936). A role represents the dynamic aspect of a status where individuals put the rights and duties which constitute a particular status into effect. Obviously roles and statuses are quite interdependent, there being no statuses without roles or roles without statuses (Davis, 1949, and Gordon, 1966).

The basic notion underlying Role Theory is that people interact according to learned expectations of behavior. This represents the individualized side of Role Theory which is of greatest interest to psychologists, counselors and other students of disability. Whereas the rights and duties attributed to statuses are generally well understood, role expectations are not as well understood. This seems attributable to the fact that there are many many more roles than statuses to learn and that people are exposed to differential socialization experiences for role learning.

The fact that individuals enact roles in different ways is not completely understood but seems attributable to a number of factors: First is that people are exposed to an unequal number of roles, which influences the knowledge of role expectations; Second, people learn role expectations with a relative degree of accuracy, depending primarily on the relative teaching abilities of significant role models; Third, people possess differential role-taking skills, dependent on learning and heredity and constitution; Finally, role enactment is influenced by unknown factors, "X" if you will, such as motivation or personality.

Related to successful role enactment is the concept of role reciprocity (Sarbin, 1954). This is the construct that every role is closely interwoven with one or more others, e.g. girl-woman, father-son, winner-loser and so on. It is believed therefore that people must understand role reciprocity if they are to accurately act out individual roles. In a general frame of reference, it might be argued that the most successful people in life are those who accurately know the expectations for the greatest number of roles, have the most outstanding role skills and the greatest drive to engage in role taking activities.

In terms of disability, it has been hypothesized that persons primarily enact roles according to their expectations, or role set, for and about the so-called "sick-role" (Gordon, 1966). Parsons (1951) believed that Role Theory affords an ideal model for evaluating the reciprocal interaction of disabled and nondisabled persons. In Parson's view, the major dyadic relationships influencing disability roles are between the physician and the patient and the patient and his family. Parsons (1951) goes on to state that these relationships must be viewed in terms of four behavioral presumptions of the sick role. First is the presumption that sick persons are exempt from social responsibility. Second is the presumption that the sick person cannot be expected to take care of himself. Illness or disability produces incapacity and consequently limits or inhibits the performance of routine duties. In this sense the sick person is viewed as incompetent, and not accountable for his actions. That is, he is in a condition that must be cared for. Parson's third behavioral presumption is that sick persons should wish to get well because health is viewed as necessary for the optimal performance of most important life tasks. Fourth, there is the presumption that society demands that sick persons should seek medical advice and cooperate with medical experts.

A psychological construct that is closely related to Parsons' behavioral presumptions about the sick role is that of "the requirement of mourning" developed by Borker, Wright and Gonick (1946) and Wright (1955). They feel that there is an expectation or demand made on disabled persons to act sick, like it or not, for a time following disablement. This expectation, to be depressed over his loss of functionality and to brood or mourn, is believed to be almost universally imposed on the disabled person. The role demands represented by the "requirement of mourning" can be considered to be infectious and applicable to nearly all disabled and nondisabled persons. On the part of the disabled persons, mourning has frequently been observed, especially closely after disablement, along with such related affective dimensions as self-devaluation and spread or the generalization of dysfunctional anxiety (Wright, 1960). Significant others, that is, those persons who are closest to and psychologically most important to the disabled also experience the "mourning" response in what can be viewed as a sympathetic response due to a case of overidentification with the disabled person. Finally, some nondisabled persons who are not significant others — they may, in fact, not even personally know the disabled person — may require the disabled individual to mourn his loss because they are personally threatened by the person's medical condition or have a pathological need to feel psychologically superior.

In addition to the statements already made, Role Theory can be extended still further to explain the psychological impact of disability on so-called disabled and nondisabled individuals. In terms of the disabled themselves, it has been hypothesized that the response to disablement is quite individualized (Gordon, 1966). It has further been hypothesized (Parsons, 1958) that illness or disability disrupts established role patterns and leads to a reorganization of roles, which is also applicable to rehabilitation treatment or service which is designed to restore or maximize the person's ability to enact roles appropriately. These hypotheses have all been studied to some extent and are generally supported by research findings (McDaniel, 1969, and Wright, 1960).

As might be anticipated, given the embryonic development of a psychology of disability, not all hypotheses put forth by role theorists have been supported by research findings. For example, Parsons (1958) predicted that the severity of disability or illness would be directly related to the degree of individual psychopathology expressed by a disabled person. The conclusions of English (1968), McDaniel (1969) and Wright (1960), who have all written extended literature reviews on this topic, dispute this hypothesis.

Apart from those hypotheses, derived from Role Theory, which have or have not found support, there are many which apply to both the reciprocal disabled and nondisabled actors which simply have not been researched sufficiently to allow for definitive conclusions. It is assumed, for example, that disablement promotes a higher incidence of role conflict among the disabled and the nondisabled with whom they interact. The disabled, for example, are believed to be placed in the ambiguous situation of having to choose between acting "as if" they were healthy or sick, and the nondisabled encounter similar problems in wrestling with the question of how to treat the so-called disabled person. Related to this, it is believed, without substantiation as yet, that much of the negative interaction that has been observed as taking place between disabled and nondisabled persons, after traumatic disablement, can be ascribed to uncertainty about what are appropriate role expectations and role enactments. Theoretically, again this hypothesis has yet to be adequately tested, this explains why the disabled and nondisabled have unsatisfactory interactions and why the disabled promote "prejudice by invitation" and why the nondisabled inadvertently stigmatize the disabled (Wright, 1960). As a final example, more research needs to be forthcoming with regard to the concept of "stigma by association." This refers to the notion, developed by Olshansky (1965), that nondisabled persons, especially nonfamily members such as counselors or teachers, are often themselves victims of prejudice and devalued simply because of their interaction with the disabled.

OVERVIEW

Up to this point, the focus of this article has been on presenting in rather straight-forward terms the relative merits of four prominent and, I believe, promising personality theories as they apply to a psychology of disability. At this juncture, all the theories will be cast into a common conceptual model and briefly analyzed. The article will end after some succinct concluding remarks.

In Table 1-I the relative effects of two etiological conditions are considered, within the framework of four personality theories, as they apply to the psychological adjustment of the physically disabled. The subjective judgments that are made, in this table and in three others that follow, are solely those of the author. Evaluations made involved analysis on a five point scale: very definitely; definitely; probably; somewhat; and slightly or not at all.

TABLE 1-I

THE EFFECT OF HEREDITY AND EARLY CHILDHOOD ON THE PSYCHOLOGICAL ADJUSTMENT OF THE PHYSICALLY DISABLED

Personality Theories	(1) Heredity Influences the Psychological Adjustment of the Physically Disabled	(2) Early Childhood Education Influences the Psychological Adjustment of the Physically Disabled
Psychoanalytic Theory	Very Definitely	Very Definitely
Individual Psychology	Very Definitely	Very Definitely
Body Image Theory	Definitely	Definitely
Role Theory	Slightly or Not at All	Somewhat

The theoretical data contained in Table 1-I suggest that heredity and early childhood are believed to be very critical factors, influencing the psychological adjustment of physically disabled persons, by psychoanalytic theorists and Adlerians, while Body Theorists believe they are only critical and Role Theorists believe they are relatively inconsequential.

Conceptually these differences reflect the basic character of these theories. That is, they range on a continuum from the most pure psychological theory (psychoanalytic) to refined psychological theories (individual psychology and body image theory) to one of the most pure of sociological theories (role theory). These differences are, of course, only logical, given their historical origins. Considering that Freud and his protege Adler were medical men most active around the turn of the twentieth century, it is hardly surprising that they developed basically psychogenic theories of personality. In related fashion, Body Image Theory and Role Theory reflect the times in which they were written as well as the backgrounds of their major protagonists. Most body theorists have been psychologists, and nearly all of their work has been done since 1930. Most role theorists are sociologists or socialpsychologists, and nearly all of their work is post World War II.

The theoretical conclusions offered in Table 1-II suggest that all

TABLE 1-II

THE PSYCHOLOGICAL IMPACT OF DISABLEMENT

Personality Theories	(3) Disablement Adversely Affects the Psychological Adjustment of the Physically Disabled	(4) Disablement Adversely Affects the Psychological Adjustment of the Significant Others of the Physically Disabled
Psychoanalytic Theory	Somewhat	Somewhat
Individual Psychology	Very Definitely	Definitely
Body Image Theory	Definitely	Probably
Role Theory	Somewhat	Somewhat

the personality theories considered here believe that disablement has a negative effect on the psychological adjustment of the physically disabled. This seems not to be very important to psychoanalytic theorists and role theorists, but very important to Adlerians and body image theorists. In part, this interpretation of theory is based on the relative permanence of the personality core in early childhood according to psychoanalytic theorists and the relative optimism of role theorists in believing that adversity can be adjusted to. Because psychique per se is such a central construct in the other two theories, it is logical to predict that they believe that disablement will have a serious negative effect on personality.

The conclusions about the influence of disablement on the psychological adjustment of the nondisabled significant others of the disabled is fairly consistent with the preceeding interpretations. Because the people affected are secondary figures, however, the effects should not be as great.

The construct examined in Table 1-III (5) is related to the construct previously examined in Table 1-II (3). The difference lies in the fact that the first analysis focuses on the psychological impact of disablement on the disabled person's interpersonal adjustment, while the second considers the sociological impact of

TABLE 1-III
THE SOCIOLOGICAL IMPACT OF DISABLEMENT

Personality Theories	(5) Disablement Adversely Affects the Life Style of the Physically Disabled	(6) Disablement Adversely Affects the Life Style of the Significant Others of the Physically Disabled	(7) Disablement Results in Stigmatization of the Physically Disabled
Psychoanalytic Theory	Definitely	Definitely	Very Definitely
Individual Psychology	Very Definitely	Very Definitely	Very Definitely
Body Image Theory	Definitely	Probably	Probably
Role Theory	Definitely	Definitely	Somewhat

disablement on the disabled person's life style, i.e. how one lives his life, where and doing what with whom. A core component of "life style" is the notion that an individual's subjective and objective life chances are adversely changed by traumatic setbacks such as disablement (English, 1968).

In regard to these two dimensions, proponents of two personality systems, psychoanalytic theory and role theory, would seem to be prepared to argue that "disablement" does greater damage to a disabled person objectively — sociologically — than it does subjectively — psychologically. Proponents of two other theories, Adlerians and Body Image Theorists, would seem not to see clear distinctions in the psychological and sociological consequences of disablement for disabled persons, while viewing the general impact as more handicapping then would Freudians or Role Theorists.

These theoretical conclusions are substantially the same when the relative psychological and sociological consequences of disablement are considered as they might apply to disabled persons' nondisabled "significant others." An examination of Table 1-II (4) and Table 1-III (6) reflects the attitude on the part of psychoanalytic theorists and role theorists that disablement is a more handicapping condition (Hamilton, 1948) sociologically than psychologically. Body Image theorists view the impact as consistent, although individual psychologists might believe that disablement realistically affects the life styles of the disabled person's able-bodied friends and family more than it affects these significant persons psychologically.

These theoretical conclusions are relatively consistent with empirical data (English, 1968, McDaniel, 1969, and Wright, 1960) and may perhaps best be explained by two factors. First is a belief in the relative stability or permanence of personality beyond the most formative preschool years. Second is a belief that life style and socio-economic statuses are somewhat tenous realities which are indeed subject to change by major events, both good and bad. Comparatively then, it seems that psychological conditions are somewhat more stable or permanent than are sociological conditions.

One additional construct has relevance for a discussion of the sociological impact of disablement according to personality

This is the notion that disablement contributes to the stigmatization of physically disabled persons (Table 1-III, 7). Each of the four personality theories considered would appear to see some link between disablement and stigmatization, but only Freudian and Adlerian theorists seem likely to see the relationship as very substantial.

Assuming this theoretical analysis is accurate, it may best be attributed to the basic assumptions that each of these theories makes with regard to the nature of man. It is generally conceded (Hall and Lindzey, 1957) that psychoanalytic and Adlerian personality theorists take a dim view of man and his basic motivations for interpersonal interactions. These theories tend to portray man as basically hedonistic and self-oriented with definite needs to dominate others. In contrast, most body theorists would seem to hold a fairly neutral to neutral-negative view of man, while most role theorists have the attitude that man's character is basically neutral to neutral-positive.

The last set of constructs to be considered in a general conceptual model, as they relate to a psychology of disability, have to do with the rehabilitation of the physically disabled, their significant others and the liklihood of reducing stigma towards physically disabled persons. The theoretical conclusions which relate to these dimensions are presented in Table 1-IV (8, 9, 10, 11, 12).

The conclusions presented in Table 1-IV (8) clearly suggest that physically disabled persons can recover from the adverse psychological effects of disablement. Individual psychologists would be most likely to be pessimistic in this regard, given the centrality of "organic inferiority" in their theory, while role theorists would be most optimistic because of their far greater emphasis on social causality. The presumption of all four theories, however, is that personality development is relatively complete at an early age, generally well before disablement occurs. All four theories would further presume that, while disablement may force a psychological setback, it is very unlikely to lead to a total personality change. Finally, all four theories, to some degree, place a considerable degree of confidence in counseling and psychotherapy and in therapeutic environmental manipulation. In this sense, they all

TABLE 1-IV

THE PROGNOSIS FOR REHABILITATIVE TREATMENT
AND ATTITUDE CHANGE

Personality Theories	(8) Physically Disabled Persons Can Recover from Adverse Psychological Effects of Disablement	(9) The Significant Others of the Disabled Can Recover from the Adverse Psychological Effects of Disablement	(10) Physically Disabled Persons Can Recover from the Adverse Sociological Effects of Disablement	(11) Significant Others of the Disabled Can Recover from the Adverse Sociological Effects of Disablement	(12) Stigma Towards the Physically Disabled Can be Reduced
Psychoanalytic Theory	Probably	Definitely	Somewhat	Probably	Slightly or not at all
Individual Psychology	Somewhat	Definitely	Somewhat	Probably	Slightly or not at all
Body Image Theory	Probably	Probably	Probably	Probably	Somewhat
Role Theory	Very Definitely	Very Definitely	Definitely	Very Definitely	Probably

believe that personality is malleable and that psychological adjustment can be improved.

Consistent with earlier conclusions on the impact of disablement, Table 1-IV (9) suggests a more positive prognosis for recovery from the psychological effects of disablement for significant others than for the disabled themselves. The differences between the theories may best be attributable to their differential belief about the nature of man and the differential commitment people have to preserve interpersonal relationships and to help each other. Because psychoanalytic and Adlerian theorists believe man is basically motivated by self gain, their judgment that the psychological effects of disablement for nondisabled persons will be slight is absolute. In contrast, the similar conclusion by role theorists is conditional and requires qualification. Their conviction that significant others will rebound from the negative effects of disablement is based on the same conviction for the disabled themselves. These roles are symbiotic and, because they are, most role theorists would argue that, where physically disabled persons do not psychologically recover from the adverse effects of disablement, their significant others probably will not either.

The theoretical conclusions presented in Table 1-IV (10, 11) regarding the prognosis for recovering from the sociological effects of disablement by the disabled and their significant others is consistent with the data presented in Table 1-III (5 and 6) regarding the sociological impact of disablement. The prognosis is generally more pessimistic for recovering from the sociological effects than the psychological effects of disablement, as presented in Table 1-IV (8 and 9). As before, we see more optimism among the newer and more sociological theories, Body Theory and Role Theory.

Finally, Table 1-IV (12) presents conclusions about the chances of reducing stigma towards physically disabled persons. As would be expected, it was suggested that psychoanalytic and Adlerian theorists would be very pessimistic about changing negative attitudes towards disabled persons, while Body and Role theorists would hold some medium degree of optimism.

CONCLUDING REMARKS

In this theoretical article, attention has been paid to the relative value of four personality theories for explaining psychological reactions to physical disability. The theories considered (psychoanalytic, individual psychology, body image and social role) are not exhaustive, but do appear to be among the most promising for explaining a general psychology of disability. Similarly, the conclusions reached in this article should be considered as tentative, challengeable, and hypothesis-generating in nature. Last, although the article's contents focused on physical disability, it appears to have substantial relevance to other disability groups.

All of the theories considered here, but especially those developed by Freud and Adler, can be faulted for having very little meaningful empirical research to back them. In fact, on some issues their hypotheses are in direct conflict with research findings. For example, all the theories suggest that disablement has a slight to profound impact on psychological adjustment, but several fairly exhaustive literature reviews suggest that there are few if any real personality differences between disabled and nondisabled persons (English, 1968, McDaniel, 1969, and Wright, 1960).

Early in this article certain positive attributes of each theory were presented. However each has certain liabilities as well as systems to comprehensively relate to a psychology of disability. Psychoanalytic theory seems to place a disproportional emphasis on sex, heredity, early childhood and the negative side of man. Some of these same criticisms appear applicable to Individual Psychology, regarding overemphasis on heredity, early childhood and projecting a very pessimistic image of man. Moreover, Adlerian theorists can be faulted for indiscriminately applying some concepts, e.g. compensation and inferiority (McDaniel, 1969)

The most damaging criticisms applicable to Body Image Theory seem to relate to a general feeling that it is too oblique and lacks comprehensiveness to such an extent that it may not be a theory at all. Furthermore, it may be faulted for failure to clearly discriminate the constructs of body image and self-concept. Finally, role theory seems inadequate to completely explain a psychology of disability because it is too sociological and does not attribute enough importance to personality and psychological variables.

At the present time Role Theory seems to have a slight edge over the other three theories, but what is obviously needed is more research, both theoretical and empirical, on the application of theory to a developing psychology of disability. It is, frankly, appalling that rehabilitationists have not made more use of theory in their efforts to assist the disabled. Hopefully this article will ameliorate this situation to some degree.

DISCUSSION QUESTIONS

1. What concepts presented in this chapter do you disagree with, if any?
2. Discuss your theory of adjustment to physical disability.

REFERENCES AND SUGGESTED READING

Adler, A. The Practice and Theory of Individual Psychology. New York, Harcourt-Brace, 1927.

Abel, T. A. Figure drawing and facial disfigurement. Am J Orthopsychiatry, 23:253-264, 1954.

Barker, R., Wright, B. and Gonick, M. Adjustment to Physical Handicaps and Illness: A Survey of the Social Psychology of Physique and Disability. New York, Social Science Research Council, 1946.

Cleveland, S. E. Body image changes associated with personality reorganization. J Consult Psychol, 24:256-261, 196.

Davis, K. Human Society. New York, MacMillan Co., 1949.

English, R. W. Assessment of Change in the Personal-Social Self-Perceptions of Vocational Rehabilitation Clients. Unpublished doctoral dissertation, University of Wisconsin, Madison, 1968.

English, R. W. Correlates of Stigma Towards Physically Disabled Persons. Rehabilitation Research and Practice Review (Accepted for publication, Fall, 1971).

English, R. W. and Oberle, J. B. Toward the development of new methodology for examining attitudes toward disabled persons. Rehabil Counsel Bull 15:88-96, 1971.

Fisher, S. and Cleveland, S. E. Body Image and Personality. New York, Dover Publications, Inc., 1968.

Gordon, G. Role Theory and Illness. New Haven, Conn., College and University Press Services, Inc., 1966.

Hall, C. S. and Lindzey, G. Theories of Personality. New York, John Wiley and Sons, 1957.

Kohler, W. Gestalt Psychology. New York, Mentor, 1947.

Linton, R. The Study of Man. New York, Appleton-Century-Crofts Co., 1936, pp. 113-114.

McDaniel, J. W. Physical Disability and Human Behavior. New York, Pergamon Press, 1969.

Oshansky, S. S. Stigma: Its meaning and some of its problems for vocational rehabilitation agencies. Rehabil Lit, 26:71-74, 1965.

Parsons, T. The Social System. Glencoe, Illinois, The Free Press, 1951.

Parsons, T. Definitions of health and illness in the light of American values and social structure. In E. G. Jaco (Ed.) Patients, Physicians and Illness. Glencoe, Illinois, The Free Press, 1958. Chapter 20, pp. 165-187.

Popper, J. M. Motivational and social factors in children's perception of height. Doctoral dissertation, Stanford University. Palo Alto, California, 1957.

Sarbin, T. R. Role theory. In G. Lindzey (Ed.) Handbook of Social Psychology. Cambridge, Massachusetts, Addison-Wesley Publishing Co., 1954, p. 223.

Schilder, P. The Image and Appearance of the Human Body. New York, John Wiley and Sons, 1950.

Silversetin, A. B. and Robinson, H. A. The representation of orthopedic disability in children's figure drawings. J Consult Clin Psychol, 20:333, 1956.

Wapner, S. and Werner, H. (Ed.) The Body Percept. New York, Random House, 1965.

Witkin, H. A., Lewis, H. B., Hertzman, M., Machover, K., Meissner, P. B. and Wapner, S. Personality through Perception. New York Harper and Row, 1954.

Wright, B. Physical Disability: A Psychological Approach. New York, Harper and Row, 1960.

Wright, B. The period of mourning in chronic illness. In R. Harrower (Ed.) Medical and Psychological Teamwork in the Care of the Chronically Ill. Springfield, Thomas, 1955.

Yuker, H. E., Block, J. R. and Younng, J. H. The Measurement of Attitudes Toward Disabled Persons. Human Resources Center, Albertson, New York, 1966.

Chapter 2

THE EPILEPTIC

    Case Number One
    Case Number Two
    Case Number Three
    Summary
    Discussion Questions
    Suggested Reading

SINCE the beginning of the history of mankind, the fear of the unknown has plagued peoples of the world. The disability known as "Epilepsy" has been one of those unknown, unexplainable afflictions.

At one time in history, it was believed that the individual who had epilepsy was "afflicted" or "possessed by evil spirits." Later on, the idea appeared that the individual was being punished for "sins, or wrong doings" of his parents or ancestors. Still later, it was commonly thought that the condition was inherited from the parents. There are still those in society who think some of the reasons listed above are the cause of epilepsy. When a parent discovered that his child appeared to have epilepsy, the immediate reaction was to think of how the child would be treated, or how the neighbors and friends would look upon the family. Families, therefore, have tried to keep the fact hidden from all. Children were withdrawn from school; if not, many times school authorities would request that they be taken out. Children in the neighborhood were told not to play with them. Many of these boys and girls became inmates of state and county institutions because their parents did not know what else to do for them.

In reference to rehabilitation, with the research and the increased knowledge of medication to control seizures, it would appear that rehabilitation should be accomplished with considerable results. However, there is still a great deal of confusion in the minds of many in regard to epilepsy. Since there are many types, with varying degrees of severity, some of which seem to be easier to control than others, there is much research still to be accomplished.

It is very difficult to determine the number of individuals who are subject to epilepsy because there are still many persons who do not wish to divulge the fact that they have seizures. If the broader classification under the general title of "convulsive disorder" would be used, a much greater number of cases would be found. It is believed by many that the term "convulsive disorder" would be much more desirable and would enable the rehabilitation counselor to secure greater results. The stigma and fear of the term "epilepsy" would no longer automatically close the door on employment opportunities.

In the past, we have heard of the "epileptic personality." In studying and working with individuals, we have encountered in the older adults a great deal of hostility. As we realize how the environment has treated them from the time it was known that they were subject to epileptic seizures, we begin to understand why many of them have become embittered. The reaction would almost be normal under this situation.

In thinking of rehabilitation services for this group, it must be recognized that there are many factors that contribute to the difficulty of achieving a suitable placement for these individuals. The first goal for the rehabilitation service is to be able to reach the person who has the disability. In order to accomplish this, the services, and what they may be able to help the individual to accomplish, must become more widely known. The program may be able to provide this information and knowledge through use of the news media, through local appearances before groups such as service clubs, classes in school, medical societies, etc. A major source of help that is developing in the United States is "The Epilepsy Foundation of America" and its state and local affiliates. One of the main purposes of this organization is to provide knowledge and information to all, so the problem of epilepsy may be better understood and, consequently, the individual allowed to take his rightful place in society.

There also have been a number of developments in the

rehabilitation field that should be of great benefit to the person with this disability. In the medical field, intensive research is being carried on. The field of neurology is doing more research in reference to the cause and treatment of this disorder.

In the vocational area, the development of workshops and the concept of performance evaluation is important.

In the psychological aspect, the concept of "behavior modification" has real meaning for epilepsy.

In other important areas, there have been many developments that help in the rehabilitation process in the past few years. Many states have developed procedures by which the issuance of drivers licenses to individuals with a history of seizures is made. This usually is handled by a medical board to review the recency of seizures and the medication being used to control the seizures. It generally requires substantiation of the application by a medical report. The ability to drive with a license is a moral boost for the epileptic. It also enables the counselor to search for jobs that are in outlying areas where there may be no transportation system.

The matter of securing insurance is also an area in which progress is being made. There are companies that have become interested in insuring the handicapped and some companies have developed a special insuring program for the epileptic.

With increased knowledge and techniques, it is believed that rehabilitation counselors should have more ability to provide needed services to this disabled group.

The formal rehabilitation process should provide the following services to a person who is referred to them:
1. An adequate diagnosis, consisting of:
    (a) Medical evaluation.
    (b) Psychological evaluation.
    (c) Social evaluation.
    (d) Work evaluation.
2. Counseling, consisting of:
    (a) Interpretation of the information.
    (b) Planning with client for the determination of a suitable vocational objective.
3. Implementation of a plan, consisting of the following:
    (a) Services needed.

(b) Location of training facility or suitable job placement.
(c) Length of time needed to achieve the plan.
(d) Provision of coordination of services needed in order to achieve goal.
(e) Continual review and evaluation during the training period.
(f) Follow-up services after placement to insure job suitability and satisfaction.

The rehabilitation process has been developed to provide needed services on an individual basis. The services are provided by the rehabilitation program through a staff person usually known as a counselor. The success of a program for an individual will depend on the relationship between the client and the counselor. In order to work with clients with this particular disability, the counselor must have considerable knowledge in reference to the disability, the pressures and influences that have been brought to bear on the client, the method of dealing with all these factors that the client has followed, the antagonism and hostilities that are a part of the attitude of the client, and last, the counselor must deal with the client in a practical, realistic way. The counselor who is assigned to work with a client who is subject to seizures must be aware that this is a particular challenge to his counseling ability and be willing to accept this challenge. The rewards to the counselor will be forthcoming when clients who have never worked are trained and able to work, when a father and mother of a client come to see him and thank him for what has been accomplished for their son or daughter and in many other intangible ways.

Caution must be expressed to the counselor who may have great expectations in this field. There are still many in our society who believe that a person subject to seizures should be institutionalized, or that they should not be in school, or that they are unable to work. Very recently a training school representative said to a rehabilitation staff, they would accept all disabilities for training as draftsmen, with the exception of a person with epilepsy.

Many times the client or members of his family may ask the counselor the question, "What kind of job can a person with epilepsy do?" The answer to this question is complicated by a number of factors. The client must recognize that there is no particular job that is best for all clients. Each case must be carefully considered. The differences in interests, in abilities, in the degree of disability, all must help in the client's decision. At one time, it was believed that a person who had seizures should not work in anything but a safe job. Today, with adequate control, jobs near moving equipment, on assembly lines, up on scaffolds, etc., are being done by people who ten or fifteen years ago would have to be doing something different. Of course, it must be recognized there are some positions which still will not accept a person for employment. Such jobs as airplane piloting. It would not be practical to think in terms of putting a person with epilepsy into training to become a pilot.

It should be pointed out that in many cases epilepsy may not make the person eligible for the rehabilitation program. An individual whose seizures are well controlled, and who has a trade, or who is well trained in an occupational skill, and who is working because of his skills, would not meet the second requirement; namely, "there must be a substantial obstacle to employment" as a result of the disability. Many people have believed the individual with epilepsy should be eligible because of the "stigma" attached to epilepsy. If he is not working, few rehabilitation agencies will not accept the person as a client. This is because it is well known that job placement will be very difficult, even if the client is well trained. This, again, illustrates the need for more education and knowledge to society and especially for the contact with employers. There are many obstacles to be overcome, but there is much help coming to assist the counselor who is willing to work in this field.

The expanding programs of The American Foundation of Epilepsy, the development of performance evaluations, work adjustment training, increasing research in the field of medicine, the passage of the Developmental Disabilities Act, in some localities the development of Epi-Hab Workshops and the overall interest and desire of society to provide help for the disabled are all to be considered on the counselor's side. In order to take advantage of all these developments, the rehabilitation program and the counselor must become involved. The services must be made available, and in order to help increase community knowledge, counselors are being invited to become participants in these developments. If the counselor stands on the side lines and says, "I'm here to serve those you wish to send," the services will not be used to the extent they should.

The combined efforts of all groups working in the field of epilepsy must be directed toward increasing the knowledge of employers. They are, in most cases, the key to the rehabilitation of the epileptic. Unless a job is realized after the services are provided, the accomplishment of the services is worth very little. This is true for all our members of society. We see many well-trained individuals working in fields where only minimal training is required. This is a waste of human resources.

In order to open up jobs, personnel people need to be contacted and perhaps even used in an advisory capacity. Counseling is important because plans must be based on practical information. The counselor might well be the person to develop and establish a counseling and advisory committee from the industrial section of the community. This committee would also help to promote increased knowledge to employers. There are many advantages which might be gained by having or developing such a committee to help in reference to the furthering of jobs for the epileptic.

In order to achieve suitable employment for the young person who is referred for rehabilitation services, it is well to recognize that an education and special training will better prepare an individual to seek employment. The individual who has a high school education is usually chosen for a position in a company or establishment over the individual who lacks a high school diploma. If an individual has not finished his high school education, it is possible to take a General Educational Development test and secure a high school equivalency certificate in lieu of a high school diploma. This will help to open some employment opportunities, although there will still need to be the specialized training for a specific job or occupation.

Skills often will overcome some of the hesitancy which the employer may have because of the fear or lack of knowledge of epilepsy.

The rehabilitation counselor or agency that is located in the vicinity where a medical facility, which may sponsor an epilepsy clinic, is very fortunate. The staff of such a clinic is generally very interested in working closely with the rehabilitation program. They will provide consultation on cases, training for the counselors on the problem of epilepsy, training for the medical consultants, and help in any other way that will be beneficial to the client. They provide for the counselors to receive the reports on each individual referred to them for evaluation and medication. This has been found to be a resource of very great value and sometimes is overlooked by both the agency and the staff.

The following cases are presented to show various ways in which the rehabilitation program may serve those with the disability of epilepsy. The cases are not discussed as being a model or for any other reason than to present some facts on what may be accomplished by the individual who wishes to make use of resources to help him help himself.

CASE NUMBER ONE

Referral date — July 17, 1971.
Referred by high school nurse.
White, male, 18 years of age.
High school graduate, completed high school in June.
Lives with maternal grandparents.
No other children in the home.
Parents divorced. No brothers or sisters.

Disability — epileptic seizures, grand mal — under medication.
Seizures well controlled.
Report from medical clinic where his case is being followed.
Appears to be well adjusted, but anxious about the future.

Test results:
    Intelligence — high average.
    Interests — clerical and scientific were highest areas of interest.
            Personnel and social fields were low.
    Aptitude — scientific, clerical.

Medical consultant's report:
    Seizures well controlled. No other medical problems.
Work experience: Part time, only. Nothing related to what he would like to do.

Total evaluation indicated several fields in which interest and aptitude were such that chances of success were good.

Client decided on an introductory course in accounting. This was tentative. Client brought his grandmother to the office to meet the counselor and discuss the tentative plan. The grandmother expressed interest in the method used in helping the client arrive at the decision to take training in the field of accounting. When it was explained, the question was asked if the client could get a job in this field, or would his disability bar him from entering the employment field. After receiving assurance that this field would offer an opportunity for employment, the final decision was made.

Plan development:

Client chose a private business school. Maintenance, transportation and supplies were to be provided by the grandparents. The rehabilitation program will provide tuition for the course. The course is to last for a period of twelve months. Training started in September. Progress was satisfactory through five months. In February, a brief time out to visit the medical clinic to check on medication. Training resumed after two weeks. Progress continues to be satisfactory.

Training completed in October. Training agency placed client in a position with a small hotel. Client liked job. Employer was well pleased with work of client. No problems with epilepsy. Three month follow-up before closure. Client working and satisfied with job. Employer still pleased. Case closed.

Six months later client came to office to visit with counselor. Had received an offer of employment with a hotel chain. Was of the opinion he should take it, because the chances of advancement were much greater than where he was working. The question of pressure was discussed in reference to the larger company. The possibility of moving from Denver was also discussed with the counselor. The client left with instructions to let the counselor know what his decision was. Two days later he phoned to say he was accepting the new job. Two months later he phoned to report he was doing well. No further contacts.

CASE NUMBER TWO

Referral date — October 7, 1972.
Made his own appointment over the phone.
Had heard of the program over a local radio station.
White, male, single, 46 years of age.

Never been married, no dependents.
Lived alone in a small apartment.
Had a high school education.
Trained as a machinist and currently working.
Epilepsy – nocturnal seizures, only, according to his report.
Program explained to him by counselor.
Discussion centered on the eligibility requirements for the vocational rehabilitation program. Client did not wish to be declared as not meeting the requirements for service. He was of the opinion rehabilitation should provide some social and recreational outlets for clients. Certain suggestions were made to him in order that he might have some social contacts. The Colorado Epilepsy Association was discussed, as was the possibility of enrolling in night classes at the Denver Emily Griffith Opportunity School. The value of joining a church group was also discussed. It was pointed out to the applicant that the rehabilitation program did not provide purely recreational or social activities.

The applicant left the office and was later visited with several times at Colorado Epilepsy Association meetings. At first, there appeared to be a certain amount of hostility towards the counselor and the agency, but as the individual became more involved, this hostility appeared to lessen and he is currently on very friendly terms with the counselor and has spoken in favor of the rehabilitation program in two meetings.

CASE NUMBER THREE

Referral date – February 14, 1973.
Referred by Colorado State Employment Service.
White, female, 35 years of age.
High school graduate, no other special training.
Divorced, no dependents.
Parents now providing for her living expenses.
Referred by employment services because she is having trouble with seizures and is untrained.

Program explained to applicant and following this interview, an appointment was made for a general medical examination and also an appointment was made for testing at the State Employment Service.

Medical report received:
Recommendation for an evaluation at Epilepsy Clinic for more adequate control of seizures. Medical consultant concurred with this

recommendation.
Appointment made for client at Epilepsy Clinic.
Test scores received from the Employment Service.
High in clerical and sales.
Verbal ability — high average.
Results discussed with client.
Her decision was to take training in the stenographic field.
This training program was not to begin until clearance received from the Epilepsy Clinic.
Report received and training started. Nine-month training course completed without further problems.
Placement presented a problem.
Client finally decided to try for a State Civil Service position. Filed an application.
Counselor was called in reference to her disability.
Finally accepted after a medical report was forwarded to them stating that her seizures were controlled by medication.
Client was placed on a job as a result of an examination and is continuing to function satisfactorily on the job.
Client's case closed after 90-day follow-up period.

SUMMARY

This has been a brief description of the rehabilitation program, the needs and challenges, to provide the services to the person who has seizures, or is known as an epileptic.

One of the most important needs is to increase the knowledge and education of all sectors of our society in reference to this disability.

The rehabilitation process is briefly outlined. Emphasis is placed on the developments that have taken place in the last few years that should help in the rehabilitation of the epileptic.

The importance of the counselor, the knowledge, the understanding and the challenge facing this position are discussed in a very limited way.

This chapter is not intended to provide more than a preliminary glimpse of the rehabilitation program and the attempt that is being made to secure all needed services for those with this particular disability.

DISCUSSION QUESTIONS

1. What type of medical diagnostic information is essential in rehabilitation work with the epileptic?
2. What is the usual medication epileptics must take to control seizure problems and how does the effect of such medication relate to work?
3. Discuss whether or not there exists such a phenomenon as "the epileptic personality"?

SUGGESTED READING

Bagley, C. The social psychology of the child with epilepsy. London, Routledge & Kegan, Paul, 1971.

Barkemeyer, L.E. Selling of the employer. In Total rehabilitation of the epileptic – gateway to employment. Washington, D.C., U.S. Department of Health, Education, and Welfare, 1962.

Barrow, L. and Fabing, D. Epilepsy and the law. (2nd Ed.), New York, Harper & Row, 1966.

Baus, G.J., Letson, L.L., and Russell, E. Group sessions for parents of children with epilepsy. J Ped, 52:270-273, 1958.

Caveness, W.J., Merrit, W.H., and Gallup, G.H. A survey of public attitudes toward epilepsy in 1969 with an indication in trends over the past twenty years. Epilepsia. 10:429-440, 1969.

Defries, A. and Browder, S. Group therapy with epileptic children and their mothers. Bull N Y Acad Med. 28:235-240, 1952.

Frank, D.S. The multi-troubled jobseeker: The case of the jobless worker with a convulsive disorder. Washington, D.C., The Epilepsy Foundation, 1967.

Frank, D.S. Three cities job clinic and services system manual. Washington, D.C. The Epilepsy Foundation, 1969.

Gastaut, H. et.al. Epilepsy and heredity. Epilepsia. 10:3-96, 1969.

Goldin, G.J., Perry, S.L., Margolin, K.L., Stotsky, B.A., and Foster, J.C. The rehabilitation of the young epileptic. Lexington, Mass., D.C. Health, 1971.

Gruneberg, S. and Pond, D.A. Conduct disorders in epileptic children. J Neurol Neurosurg Psychiatry, 20:65-68, 1957.

Guerrant, J.J., Anderson, W., Fisher, A., Weinstein, M.R., Jaros, R.M., and Deskins, A. Personality in epilepsy. Springfield, Thomas, 1962.

Hardy, R.E. and Cull, J.G. Severe Disabilities: Social and Rehabilitation Approaches. Springfield, Thomas, 1974.

Kleck, R. Self Disclosure Patterns Among Epileptics. Hanover, New Hampshire,

Dartmouth College, 1968.

Kram, C. Epilepsy in children and youth. In W.M. Cruickshank, (Ed.), Psychology of Exceptional Children and Youth, (2nd ed.). Englewood Cliffs, Prentice-Hall, 1963.

Livingston, S. Comprehensive Management of Epilepsy in Infancy, Childhood and Adolescence. Springfield, Thomas, 1972.

Richard, T., Triandia, H., and Patterson, C. Indices of employer prejudice toward disabled applicants. J Appl Psychol, 47:52-55, 1963.

Sands, H. Changing Employment Policies and Attitudes Towards Persons with Epilepsy. Washington, D.C., Epilepsy Association of America, 1970.

Scmidt, R.P. and Wilder, B.J. Epilepsy. Philadelphia, F.A. Davis Company, 1968.

Temkin, O. The Falling Sickness (2nd ed.) Baltimore, Johns Hopkins Press, 1971.

Tizard, B, The personality of epileptics: A discussion of the evidence. Psychology Bulletin, 59:196-210, 1962.

Chapter 3

CASE STUDY SPINAL CORD INJURY

Discussion Questions
Suggested Reading

THIS twenty-eight year old married female referred herself to the agency through a county health nurse assigned to home nursing care in a rural area of Alabama. The public health nurse indicated to the counselor by phone that the client was a "very bright and very cheerful little lady who is paralyzed in all four extremities."

The counselor's first contact with the client was a home visit requiring a trip of some forty-five miles from the counselor's office. Cats and dogs of every description met the counselor on the carport, at the door and inside the house. The client was sitting upright in a wheelchair with a plywood strip across the wheelchair arms which contained a book and periodically one or two cats. After the introductions, the client indicated that she was alone and would spend the afternoon as she normally did with her "pets" which consisted of five dogs, eight cats and two birds.

The client was neatly dressed in slacks and over-blouse with socks and loafers; however, the most significant aspect of her appearance was her smile. Her speech pattern was that of an educated person and her facial expressions were very lively and appropriate. Throughout the interview, the client would occasionally interrupt the discussion to chide a wayward cat who had jumped upon the table or to humorously scold a dog who was chewing on the corner of a rug. Throughout the interview, the client was extremely still with a statue-like quality except for an occasional movement of the head. The client spoke very freely and related a good history, indicating that as the aftermath of an automobile accident at age sixteen, she had been paralyzed in all four extremities and had been unable to attend school past the ninth grade. Her medical history included extensive hospitalization in Children's Hospital under the sponsorship of Crippled Children's Service, during which time she developed a secondary disability of a polio-like nature which caused her breathing to be totally voluntary. Four surgical procedures were attempted on the client to correct the paralysis but at the approximate age of twenty-one years, all medical attempts at improvement and correction were abandoned, and the client was told that she had reached maximum improvement from surgery, physical therapy and medical treatment. The client related a history of susceptibility to throat and lung infections, which have periodically demanded hospitalization and intensive medical treatment including the use of artificial breathing apparatuses. She explained that her parents had reared her in a rural section of the state where her father farmed a small rented acreage and worked in the coal mines when work was available. The client's father has in later years developed "black lung" disease and has been retired by the mines.

As the initial interview continued, the counselor became more aware of client's speech pattern, word usage and general vocabulary, and commented on this to the client. The client eagerly demonstrated her ability to slowly turn the pages of a book on her lap board by moving her head sideways, using the rubber tip of an unsharpened pencil held between her teeth. Although she could not slide her foot along the floor nor raise it from the floor, she demonstrated her ability to pat this foot. She could also slide her left hand slowly some two inches across her lap board. The client was unable to lift her left hand or fingers but had the ability to slightly grasp with the thumb of her left hand. The client's right hand and arm had no motion and she was unable to move them in any manner. The client related that should her arms slip from her lap board, she must wait until a neighbor dropped in to replace them on the lap board. The client demonstrated her ability to nod and shake her head, but when the head was tilted backward, it was very difficult for her to bring it back to a normal position.

At this time, the counselor had no intentions of activating the case but indicated to the client the services available to handicapped persons through the agency, with a major emphasis on employment as the end result of services. The client was over-joyed and assumed that since the counselor was there, explaining the services of the agency to her, there could be no thought in his mind other than assisting her in securing some type of employment. The counselor was surprised that the client thought she could work. No forms had been completed at this time and the counselor left the client with the promise to return in two weeks. It is doubtful that the counselor fully intended to keep his promise of the second interview but the following week while visiting a local high school some eight miles from the client's residence, the counselor was confronted by the high school principal. The principal congratulated the counselor in being willing to accept such a severe case but questioned the counselor regarding rehabilitation plans for the client. It seemed the entire community, approximately four thousand people, knew the client and had a great appreciation for her cheerful personality.

During the second interview on November 21, 1971, the necessary forms were completed. By this time the counselor had been contacted by a county welfare caseworker who was amazed that the client was being accepted for services but offered her assistance, complete with medical information, social history and moral support. The caseworker's only request was that she be kept informed of the progress made with the case and that the counselor do whatever he could to encourage the client to get rid of her pets. On a routine visit the counselor had dropped by the office of the only doctor in the community. The doctor informed the counselor that accepting the client into the caseload was a cruel act, since the physician had cared for the client for a number of years, was positive that no medical treatment could improve her physical condition and felt that there was no hope of the client ever securing employment.

Also during the second interview while securing additional social information, the client told the counselor that she had been married only four years. The client's husband was also handicapped having an enucleated left eye. Some three years ago, the couple had secured a low interest loan and had built a small two bedroom brick home. The husband works for a trailer manufacturing concern and experiences periodic lay-offs. At times during the year, the husband could work only one or two days per week because of production curtailments. The client's annual medical expense was the major item in the household budget since she required hospitalization approximately twice a year for treatment of chest and lung infections. Because the family could not afford an attendant, the client's daily schedule was rather unusual. The husband reported for work at 7:00 a.m. and left the client in the bed until his lunch period. At lunch time he returned home, dressed her, fed her and established her in her wheelchair, with her book and reading materials on her lap board. Here she spent the rest of the day by herself, unless a welfare social worker, neighbor or health nurse should drop in for a brief visit. The client's parents and her husband's parents were elderly and did not visit except on rare occasions. At the time of the second interview, the only cultural aspects of the family's life revolved around occasional church attendance, occasional trips to town and very rare visits to kinspeople or by kinspeople.

As the second interview closed, the client was encouraged to take a medical form to the local physician who would complete the form and return it to the counselor as routine procedure. While the counselor was gathering the necessary medical information, the client was encouraged to think of various jobs which she might be able to do.

The medical form returned by the client's physician indicated the normal examination of a married female, 5'4" tall, weighing 100 pounds, with blood pressure 100/60, pulse rate 76, slight dyspnea, wearing a back brace for support of abdomen and back, with almost complete paralysis of all four extremities. The hematocrit was 52 with the hemoglobin being 100 percent. The physician commented that the major disability was permanent and stable and indicated that the major disability could not be improved by medical treatment. There was a recommendation for a dental examination due to poor oral hygiene and dental caries. The counselor made an appointment for a full mouth examination with the only dentist in the community and arranged for the

Case Study — Spinal Cord Injury

husband to carry the client for the appointment.

On the counselor's next trip to the community, the dentist was visited and it was indicated that the dentist had a greater than average interest in the case. From the dentist's point of view, the client's use of the pencil to turn her book pages would have to be discontinued and a rather extensive program of dental filling, cleaning and general prophylactic treatment would be necessary. After this dental care, the client would be started on a routine of proper oral hygiene. The dentist was very happy that the counselor was interested in the client and indicated that on more than one occasion, he had provided free dental treatment to the client because of the family's financial situation. The counselor was assured that the dentist would cooperate in every way possible to assist the client's rehabilitation program.

The third interview with the client occurred December 18, 1971, at the client's home. During this interview, the client's medical record was discussed along with a very realistic point-by-point coverage of the client's vocational assets and liabilities. The client was first led into a discussion of her assets which centered around her self-education; this brought to the surface the fact that the client had a basic knowledge of typing which had not been discussed previously. Emotionally, the client was very mature, very realistic without the unrealistic approach often found in quadriplegics that someday, someone would do something that would make her physically whole again. The client accepted her physical limitations but doggedly reiterated her belief that there were jobs she could do if she and the counselor were just wise enough to find them. The client was no stranger to disappointment but continued to present to the counselor the optimistic viewpoint that if the first vocational endeavor failed, she was willing to try a second, and even a third endeavor, until she was vocationally successful.

There were no family problems to be solved with this client as her husband was most agreeable that she work; he offered any assistance that he could provide toward securing employment for her. The husband volunteered the information that both he and the client had discussed in detail her physical condition before they married and married with the realization that she would be limited in a number of ways. They agreed that he would be expected to do such things as the household chores while the client would be responsible for supervising these activities by instructing him in what needed to be done around the house. The husband also indicated the love life which the couple shared had never been a point of contention with either, and that both were mutually satisfied sexually and emotionally.

The client evidenced no fear or concern for her safety while her husband worked and was content to reside alone with her pets. The husband voiced some concern that the client would be easy prey to robbery, household fires or acts of nature such as storms or hurricanes. The client chided the husband, reminding him that during the four years of their married life, none of his fears had been realized. Although she admitted she would be a bit more comfortable if she had some means of communication, she was quite willing for things to continue as they were.

The couple next entered into a discussion with the counselor surrounding her physical condition, focusing upon the minus side of the vocational ledger. During this discussion, the following facts emerged: the client lived approximately eight miles from the nearest community with her only mode of transportation being a private automobile, since the community did not sponsor bus service or taxi service. Aside from the usual retail stores, the community had three small industries: a rather large sawmill, a garment factory and a small trailer manufacturing plant. Over the years the client had built her sitting tolerance to a point where she could sit for approximately six hours, provided she wore a very good quality back and abdominal support corset with metal stays. The client was totally immobile without assistance as she could not propel her wheelchair by her own strengths. She could not operate a foot pedal with either foot, nor could she operate a knee switch usually used on industrial sewing machines. She had little grasp in either hand with no lifting ability in either arm. There was a very slight possibility that she might operate a very fluid switch with the thumb of her left hand, if her hand and arm were propped in very close proximity of the switch. She could nod or turn her head from side to side, but the adaptation of this ability to industrial use could not be envisioned at this time. The client normally wore a catheter and had worked out a routine of food intake which would regulate her bowel movements and urinary activities so that these would not be factors which would adversely affect a routine job. The client needed dental work for restoration purposes and she also needed to continue to take medication to ward off urinary tract and respiratory infections. Some method other than the pencil-in-mouth had to be determined whereby she could turn the pages of her book without causing a detrimental effect to her teeth. Because of the husband's low annual income and the client's medical needs, the client had been granted "Aid to the Permanently and Totally Disabled" through the county welfare agency. This aid entitled her to medical benefits that would assist in providing hospitalization and drugs, but would not help with dental work. Any significant income which the client might receive from working would reduce the client's $79.00 per month welfare payment and might cause her to be disqualified, not only from welfare monetary assistance, but also from the hospital and medical treatment program sponsored by the welfare department. Vocational evaluation through a rehabilitation center was out of the question because of transportation difficulties; therefore, training would of necessity take place in the client's home. Finding an individual to train the client would also pose a major problem because of the client's rural setting. No physical restoration was to be considered since the counselor had secured consultation from his district medical consultant, the family physician, and the orthopedist who last treated the client and no restoration was indicated. However, based on the couple's four years of experience with the client's recurrent respiratory infections, it was expected that the client would encounter medical problems unless an unusually good job was secured. A low income job which would not disqualify the client from welfare medical programs was considered most feasible.

The counselor, client and client's husband next entered into a discussion of various vocational objectives. The client felt sure that she could type with a pencil in her mouth and could thereby address envelopes if a method could be found of placing the envelopes in the typewriter automatically. The husband felt that the client would be very good at operating a telephone answering service, provided the switching and plugging could be done automatically, with the client being required only to talk. Various sorting jobs were discussed and jobs such as quality control inspector. No local outlet could be determined for this type of work, since the quality control done in local factories required lifting, folding or handling which the client could not perform. It was decided that outside help should be secured, and the counselor assumed the responsibility for contacting individuals in the community to secure from them suggestions as to some business the client could enter locally, some service she could provide the community or some job which presently existed that she might be able to perform.

Before the counselor left the community that day he contacted the high school principal, business education and home economics teachers and two retail merchants, asking for suggestions of a job or service that the client could provide for the community from her wheelchair at home or on-the-job. Upon returning to base, the counselor solicited the assistance of another rehabilitation counselor, who worked the same community asking that he also make contacts in behalf of the client to uncover some job which might be available to her. During the next two weeks, the second counselor made contact with two ministers and a civic organization in an attempt to secure job leads for the client. The high school principal and business education teacher secured a typewriter for the client, but the most productive use found for the typewriter was personal correspondence by the client, at night while the husband was available to change the paper and insert envelopes. The client answered a number of magazine ads relating to home-bound employment but received no beneficial information. The typewriter was soon returned to the school.

After the Christmas holidays, the two counselors compared notes and used employers in the district office vicinity as sounding boards for the various recommendations which had been made. The use of a telephone continued to repeat itself in a large number of the suggestions. The local telephone company manager was consulted about methods of telephone use, the practicality of an answering service in the area where the client lived, appliances and aids available for handicapped telephone users, and telephone rates

Case Study — Spinal Cord Injury

which would affect the client. To the surprise of everyone involved, the manager of the local telephone company took a special interest in this person and made a visit with the counselor on January 2, 1972, to the client's home. The manager spent approximately an hour talking with the client and observing her use of the pencil to turn the pages of her book. He took special interest in her wheelchair and the floor plan of the house. It was the telephone company manager's idea that a telephone solicitation operation might easily be installed with the use of one private telephone line that could also be used by the client as a social contact with people outside her home, and a warning device in case of fire, break-in or storm. He felt that installation costs and community size were impractical for establishing an answering service for the client.

The manager of the local phone company provided the counselor with names of individuals who had operated and were operating telephone solicitation operations, so that they might be contacted by the counselor to determine the number of customers necessary to support such an operation. The manager sent two technicians with the counselor on his next visit to the client's house, so that the technicians might see first-hand the power with which the client could operate a telephone and thereby, adapt a phone to the client's use. The manager also dug into his files and provided the counselor with a hard-back publication entitled "Assistive Devices for the Motionally Handicapped" which provided comprehensive information and pictures relating to various types of appliances which could be attached to telephones to overcome motion deficits in handicapped persons. The counselor, client and technicians from the phone company spent approximately an hour and one-half selecting and discarding various apparatuses to hold the telephone in a position which would be accessible to the client, allowing her to turn the telephone on and off and allowing her to dial the telephone using only the muscles in her neck as a power source. After approximately two weeks of study and investigation by the telephone technicians, the counselor was contacted and advised that they had made another trip to the client's home. The technicians had taken with them a telephone which they felt had been equipped for the client's use, but it had proved nonfunctional when her pencil kept slipping from one number to another number as she tried to operate the push-button type phone which they had developed for her. During this week January 22, 1972, the counselor assisted by a second rehabilitation counselor, had contacted local clubs, organizations and merchants. These contacts were made to determine if the client could, over an extended period of time, count on sufficient customers to make a success of a telephone solicitation operation. A number of clubs and individuals wanted to make donations of money and services toward the establishment of a business for the client. Eight clubs had agreed to have the client call their membership lists on a flat fee basis. The income from these clubs was determined to be sufficient to make the proposed business a worthwhile venture. Approximately fourteen merchants had agreed to use the services of the client as much as four times each during the next twelve months by hiring the client to call the entire listing in the local phone directory to advertise special sales and promotional campaigns for their stores.

The pencil in the client's teeth could not be expected to provide continued heavy duty use which would be necessary in the dialing of the phone for the complete telephone directory list. The local dentist was, therefore, contacted and asked to develop a suitable mouthpiece which would tolerate heavy duty use, and yet be light enough for the client to grasp with her left thumb pressed against the palm of her hand and held in such a way that by a nodding motion her mouthpiece could be placed or removed with a minimum of effort. There is no way to determine the time spent by the dentist in developing the mouthpiece for the client but when it was finished, it appeared to be a set of artificial dentures which easily slipped into and out of the client's mouth with a nod of her head. From the center of the mouthpiece extended a long stainless steel tube the size of a pencil lead which had a rubber tip on its curved end. The entire apparatus was extremely light-weight and proved most functional, comfortable and satisfactory for the client.

In late January, 1972, the counselor was joined by the telephone company manager and his chief technician for another visit to the client's home. They took with them the phone company's latest proposed adaptation of a telephone to be used by the client. This personalized telephone system completed by the phone company for the client was a standard rotary dial telephone whose dial had been made so fluid that the client could easily place her mouthpiece into the slots and move her head in a clockwise fashion, thereby dialing any desired number from zero through nine. The phone had on the left hand side of its base a long handled, very fluid toggle switch which allowed the client at her will to open and close the telephone line by the use of her left thumb. When the toggle switch was in one position, the client could receive phone calls, and by switching the toggle with her thumb, the client could place outgoing calls. An adjustable brace of the gooseneck variety was clamped to the back of the client's wheelchair (and was later adapted to the client's bed) which enabled the phone to be held at ear and mouth level for the client. Its use did not require any motion on the client's part other than a tilting of her head. This brace was ordered by the telephone company and modified to fit the client's needs. The telephone technicians had little difficulty in modifying the phone and brace to adapt to the client's needs, and fitted the telephone with an unusually long retractable cord so that the telephone could be operated from any room in the house. Throughout the investigation, evaluation and installation of the telephone, the counselor, the telephone manager and the telephone technicians were in a constant program of counseling, training and reassuring the client. Even after installation of the system, additional modifications were necessary. An amplification system was added to the client's speaker because there were times when she would forget to bring her face into the correct proximity of her telephone mouthpiece, and she could not be heard by the person whom she was calling. Also, an amplification was placed into the ear phone so that the client would have no difficulty in hearing the person with whom she was speaking.

The next problem to be dealt with was that of the client's posture because she became very tired when she operated the telephone for extended periods of time. She experienced difficulty with the prolonged movement of the head that was required to dial the phone and operate the speaker and mouthpiece of the telephone. A local orthopedic appliance company was contacted on March 14, 1972, and a very strong support corset was developed by the company which would hold the client in a comfortable position and allow her to make call after call without fatigue. As a precautionary measure, at the suggestion of the appliance company, a flotation pillow was placed in the seat of the wheelchair, which made the client even more comfortable and reduced the probability of pressure sores. The client's husband made a reel for the telephone wire so that it was neatly rolled out of the way at all times. He next made a special lap board for the telephone which kept the telephone from tilting or moving. This allowed the phone to continuously be in the same proximity to the client and could easily be reached by her, using the mouthpiece. The client's husband did some local odd jobs and secured a small folding wheelchair so that the client could continue to visit relatives, attend church services, etc., without dismantling the telephone appliances which were clamped to her heavy-duty chair. The husband then modified the lap board to accommodate a toggle-switch-operated cassette recorder because the client had difficulty remembering long or complicated messages. A local electronics firm was asked to develop a means of recording telephone conversations which the client could operate on a "need" basis. The company developed a very complicated and intricate, though compact, mechanism which could be operated by a toggle switch which would allow the client to record telephone conversations at will on a low cost cassette recorder.

The counselor approached the problem of the client's many pets by suggesting that the cats and dogs could easily damage the equipment, interrupt phone conversations by noise-making and generally jeopardizing the success of the business. It was mutually agreed that the first order of business, after the phone system was functional, was for client to use her telephone to find suitable homes for her pets. All pets were given to friends, with the exception of two birds which were placed in cages and one old dog which was placed in a suitable pen in the back yard.

It became evident that a method of publicizing the client's service would be necessary if she was to continue on a permanent basis, and the manager of the local newspaper was contacted May 15, 1972, for suggestions. He became so personally involved in the case while completing a human interest story on the client that he hired the client to solicit subscriptions for the newspaper. Solicitation of newspaper subscriptions by the client was so successful (she earned $250.00 on the newspaper subscriptions alone the first month of her operation) that she was asked October 5, 1972, to solicit newspaper subscriptions semi-annually.

The local phone company published a human interest article, complete with picture, in their monthly newsletter. The newsletter was sent to each telephone customer along with the monthly phone bill. Customers were subtly informed that the client could handle additional business and that her rates were very inexpensive. As a result of the newsletter advertisement, the client secured new customers.

Soon after the client began her business, her counselor became acutely aware of the client's breathing difficulty and felt that the recurrent respiratory infection might be in some way connected with her sleeping on a "rocking bed," which had been provided through the March of Dimes state organization. An extended period of illness for the client could cause regular customers to make other arrangements which might cause the client an appreciable loss of business. An internist, who had a special interest in respiratory problems, was contacted by the counselor for consultation regarding the rocking bed. The internist felt that the bed was outmoded and that more sophisticated equipment was available. After securing a copy of the client's hospital records from her family physician, the internist recommended the purchase of a "turtle-shell respirator." This piece of equipment was relatively simple in construction and operated on household electrical current. The state organization of the March of Dimes was contacted and the problem outlined along with the request that the organization provide whatever assistance possible. Almost by return mail the client and counselor were notified that the organization would provide the respirator. The respirator would be brought to the client's home by a technician who would install the respirator and demonstrate its use. There would be no charge for the respirator or the services of the technician. After installing the respirator, the technician taught the client's husband how it should be used and maintained. That year there was no hospitalization necessary for the client.

The client continued in the operation of her business and received an established fee from every club and organization in the community. She called members of the Lion's Club, Jaycees, Civil Defense, Methodist Men's Club, Methodist Women's Club, Band Booster's Club, Athletic Booster's Club and the local Garden Club at a fee of ten cents per call to notify the members of meetings and special events. These clubs much preferred the personal contact of the telephone because messages could be relayed from one club member to another, and the cost of ten cents per call was preferred to the expenditure of secretarial time in addressing envelopes and mailing notices, each of which required an eight-cent stamp. The client continued to promote sales by local merchants on an irregular basis although she did not rely on the income from those customers but considered their business as a bonus. The client had socially multiplied her contacts and developed new friendships far beyond any degree she could have imagined and felt a closeness to almost every family and business listed in the local telephone directory. She was known by everyone in her community.

A sampling of organizations who used her services was contacted prior to this writing and without exception, those contacted indicated that they continued to be very pleased with her service. The total cost of this rehabilitation in monetary form taking into consideration medical evaluation, dental work, telephone installation and two month's service, special adaptation and modification of telephone, dorsal support, flotation pillow, recording device, modification and cassette recorder, rocking bed, shell respirator and wheelchair, which was not offset by donations from clubs and individuals toward the client's rehabilitation, was $765.45 for the agency.

This case was as significant for the counselor as for the client. He learned the value of client motivation and attitude. He learned that individuals, organizations, clubs and agencies are most willing to help and have a collective expertise that no one person could ever acquire. A large number of people enjoy helping to solve "impossible" problems. Teamwork inside an agency is an invaluable tool when working with a "tough" case. The more difficult the case, the more self-satisfaction a counselor experiences when the case is closed, rehabilitated.

DISCUSSION QUESTIONS

1. Discuss mechanical assistive devices which increase the vocational capacity of the cord injured individual.
2. Discuss the special importance of self care by the spinal cord injured person (personal hygiene problems and prevention of decubiti ulcers, bladder and bowel control).
3. Discuss sexual function in relation to spinal cord injury.

SUGGESTED READING

Felton, J.S., Perkins, D.C. and Lewin, B.A. A Survey of Medicine and Medical Practice for the Rehabilitation Counselor. Washington, D.C., Vocational Rehabilitation Administration, U.S. Department of Health, Education, and Welfare, 1966.

Freeman, L.W. Treatment of acute spinal cord injury. General Practioner, 5:00000, 1952.

French, J.J. and Porter, R.W. Basic Research in Paraplegia. Springfield, Thomas, 1962.

Frost, A. Handbook for Paraplegics and Quadraplegics. National Paraplegia Foundation, Chicago, Wallace Press, 1964.

Hardy, R.E. and Cull, J.G. Severe Disabilities: Social and Rehabilitation Approaches. Springfield, Thomas, 1973.

Howorth, M.B., Petrie, J.G., and Bennett, George Injuries of the spine. Baltimore, The Williams and Wilkins Co., 1964.

Jousse, A.T. The management of paraplegis. Manit Med Rev, 43:383-391, 1963.

Lofquist, L.H. and Dawis, R.V. Adjustment to work – A Psychological View of Man's Problems in a Work-Oriented Society. New York, Appleton-Century-Crofts, 1969.

Rosenburg, Charlot Assistive Devices for the Handicapped. Rehabilitation Publication No. 705. Minneapolis, American Rehabilitation Foundation, 1968.

Vocational Rehabilitation Administration Guidelines for Organization and Operation of Vocational Evaluation Units: A Training Guide. Rehabilitation Service Series No. 67-50. Washington, D.C., U.S. Department of Health, Education, and Welfare, 1966.

Chapter 4

CASE STUDY OF PULMONARY CONDITION

Discussion Questions
Suggested Reading

M R. Jones is a white married male, 58 years of age, who was initially referred to our agency by a general hospital in 1970 at 51. Based on a diagnostic evaluation, he was found ineligible due to the severity of his medical condition with a vital capacity approximately 50 percent of predicted precluding work on a regular basis.

He was born and educated in the northeast, where he completed eight grades of school. He resides in his own home, which was purchased prior to onset of illness. This home is in a middle class neighborhood of a medium sized manufacturing town. He resides with his wife, two grown children and elderly in-laws. There are three other children who do not live at home. Since 1964 his wife, who is an inspector in a factory, has been largely the main support of the family. The client had initially received unemployment compensation which ran out prior to his initial referral to our agency. He was determined to be eligible for Social Security Disability Benefits in 1971 for himself and, initially, for a dependent child. Mrs. Jones has had periods of unemployment during this time interval due to her own illness which has affected the financial picture.

The client's elderly in-laws receive support from the client and his wife and are an additional financial burden. Medical costs are high for the family because of his oxygen and medication requirements. He was found ineligible for medical assistance by state welfare because of an income level above their standards even with medical costs considered.

The second referral to the Division of Vocational Rehabilitation occurred in 1971 during his third hospitalization and was made by the social service department of the Rehabilitation Hospital to the counselor assigned part-time to that facility. At this time, Mr. Jones presented a picture of a depressed individual with feelings of helplessness resulting from his disability and inability to hold employment. He felt "all-burned out." The counselor initiated efforts to evaluate at that time his overall potential for employment.

While an in-patient during this hospital admission, the client was psychologically evaluated both to assess possible degree of brain damage, as suggested by poor progress and performance, and also to assist in vocational planning. Testing involved WAIS, Rorschach and Bender Gestalt. During testing, though cooperative, little interest was shown. The client was reticent and exhibited fluctuation in concentration abilities. The personality evaluation confirmed the depression presented in the client's behavior, showing a withdrawn, passive and apathetic person extremely vulnerable to feelings of rejection. Also found was a basic immaturity leading to an inability to deal with his reactions to his problems.

With regard to organicity the only indices were slight fluctuations in concentration abilities and some tendency toward cognitive fatigue toward the end of testing. The psychologist found it difficult to assess to what degree these factors were due to his overall apathy and depression. In any case, it was felt that vocational planning should not be avoided because of possible organic involvement. Memory, judgment, abstract and perceptual motor abilities were found, during testing, to be intact and WAIS showed him to be of average intelligence (full scale IQ of 100, performance of 101 and verbal of 99).

One significant observation by the psychologist was that upon completion of session, after being told he had done well and was capable of undergoing vocational planning, the client suddenly became friendly and very animated. It was a final recommendation of this psychologist that Mr. Jones would require extensive support if any program of rehabilitation would succeed.

The client was admitted to the Rehabilitation Hospital for the third time because of increasing respiratory problems worsening to the point where he was unable to walk around the house with minimal effort, resulting in exhaustion and inability to breathe at times, even at rest. It was found that his diet had been poorly regulated. Edema of lower extremities was also present although client intermittently used diuretics. He also presented a picture of depression and of having given up. Oxygen by nasal catheter (2-3 liters per minute) was required by the client along with Digoxin and the use of intermittent positive pressure breathing. Physical examination revealed signs and symptoms of chronic bronchitis and emphysema along with Cor pulmonale with increasing decompensation secondary to the overlying emphysema. Pulmonary function studies revealed severe obstructive disease with minimal improvement after bronchodilation, large residual volume and moderately severe restriction.

During the client's three month hospitalization he underwent, along with medical therapy and psychological evaluation, other evaluative and treatment modalities in a total rehabilitative effort. These included perceptual testing by occupational therapy, physical therapy and inhalation therapy. His condition at discharge on January 18, 1972, showed the Cor pulmonale and breathing pattern improved from fair to good diaphragmatic breathing with longer expirations. He also showed a greater ability to relax and was able to ambulate with almost no limitation at a slow pace requiring only occasional support from his portable oxygen equipment. He was discharged to his private physician's care. As mentioned earlier, he was also placed in contact with a counselor from the Division of Vocational Rehabilitation. The counselor was able to obtain necessary survey material and initial medical material prior to discharge, eliminating a waiting time for information. During contacts with the client, the counselor questioned the client's motivation as well as his overall potential for benefiting from vocational rehabilitation services.

Vocationally, Mr. Jones (who was not a good reporter of job history) had held fairly steady employment since prior to World War II as a factory worker. His last six years of gainful employment involved work as a toll collector ending in 1969. Amount of time lost due to illness during his jobs was not ascertained. Factory jobs included grinding, die casting, plating and assembly. All of his previous employment had environmental factors which contributed to his condition. For example, his work as a highway toll collector left him open to changes in weather, dust and other pollutants including car and truck exhausts. Approximately six months following his leaving of the job of toll collector, the client received some type of clerical training through an anti-poverty agency program but received no typing or office machine training. At the end of the training program, he was unable to find employment. At this point in evaluation of the client's potential for rehabilitation we are confronted with an individual with questionable work tolerance and motivation, limited education, few if any transferable job skills and severe environmental restrictions. Further occupational restrictions are imposed by his need for a portable oxygen device due to related hazards and lack of employer acceptance.

Educational level (8th grade) and absence of formal job training are also handicaps to employment. Another major problem was transportation. The client, though maintaining a driver's license, had let his insurance lapse and had not driven in several years. He therefore, was dependent upon his family for transportation. His wife worked considerable distance from home and no public transportation was available.

Plans were developed in consultation between the client, Division of Vocational Rehabilitation Counselor and treating physician, as well as Rehabilitation Hospital staff, for referral to a comprehensive rehabilitation facility located one-half hour from his home by car. The counselor felt that since questions existed as to reasonable expectation of benefits from services, the client should be given the benefit of further evaluation.

In order to allow the client to participate in the evaluation at the Center, it was necessary to rent a portable oxygen supply for Mr. Jones which the counselor incorporated into an extended evaluation plan effective January 23, 1972. The client was seen by a physician at the Center and a staff social worker on January 25, 1972. It was recommended by the Division of Vocational Rehabilitation counselor and the attending physician, that the client attend evaluation on a part-time basis to determine his feasibility for part-time employment. It was also felt that the feasibility of full-time work should be explored.

At the Rehabilitation Center case conference held on January 27, 1972, the concerns of the Center over the client's use of oxygen and related problems were discussed. It was felt that client tended to use the device, in part, as a crutch. In order to resolve this question it was decided to review the matter with the attending physician as well as obtain current pulmonary function studies. It was further felt that his evaluation should be geared toward sedentary work.

The counselor informed the client that he would enter the Center on February 5, 1972 on a 12 to 3 PM basis. His family would provide his transportation. The client was placed in the work evaluation unit for a twenty-day evaluation during which time the counselor maintained contact with the client on a regular basis. The client completed his prevocational evaluation on March 8, 1972 and was assigned to the workshop for work hardening and adjustment.

During the prevocational evaluation he was found to relate positively, but minimally, to both peer group and staff. He generally did not initiate conversations. In contrast to previous contacts he appeared strongly motivated and sometimes manifested work satisfaction. Adjustment to his overall evaluation was satisfactory. He had excellent attendance even with the transportation problem.

With respect to actual performance his concentrative ability was very good. He was neat in his work area. Counting skills were high in accuracy. Mr. Jones usually demonstrated conscientiousness, but frustration tolerance was not outwardly manifested. Initiative was usually evident whether or not the client was interested in the assignment. The client was able to follow oral instructions with routine demonstration and was able to follow written instructions. The work attitude seemed realistic at that time and made possible the consideration of long range planning. Mr. Jones was reliable in connection with work activities. The client had a positive attitude when under supervision and generally accepted criticism in a passive manner.

The following results were obtained during his testing period.

Case Study of Pulmonary Condition 53

PERFORMANCE

MANUAL DEXTERITY

Purdue Pegboard (Three Trials)	Score	Percentile
Right Hand	43	19
Left Hand	40	18
Both Hands	32	15
Assembly	70	4

Vocational areas explored and evaluated were: semi-clerical, electronics, bench assembly.

TEST RESULTS

Tower Clerical	Time	Quality
Abbreviations	Below Average	Below Average
Spelling	Below Average	Below Average
Composition	Below Average	Below Average
Payroll	Below Average	Average
Record-Keeping	Below Average	Below Average

Center Clerical Tests	Time	Quality
Arithmetic Symbols	Average	Above Average
Problem Solving	Above Average	Below Average
Ruler	Average	Below Average
Credit Rating	Below Average	Above Average
Adding Machine #1	Average	Below Average
Vocabulary	Below Average	Inferior
Change Making	Average	Average

Other Tower Tests

	Time	Quality
Electronics #1*	Above Average	Inferior

*In this test he had difficulty distinquishing colors.

	Time	Quality
Electronics #2, 3, 8, 9	Average	Above Average

WORK SAMPLES

Bench Assembly	Industrial Norms. r/c	Client Output $/hr.
Terminal Nut Assembly	.55	2.02
Small Bracket Assembly	.49	1.48
Ramset Spring Assembly	.26	1.18
Black Detent Assembly	.24	1.06

Packaging

12 Pop Rivets	.72	.70

In terms of qualitative standards the client's work would, if he has the physical tolerance, measure up to the requisites of the labor market.

Based on the prevailing hourly wage of $1.60, the client averaged $1.25 per hour.

STANDARDIZED TEST RESULTS

Otis Quick-Scoring Mental Ability Test

Raw Score: 14   I.Q. 72

Mechanical Comprehension Test (Form AA)

Total Score: 16   Percentile Rank: 4   Table: III - unskilled

Kuder Preference Record (Vocational Forms CH and CM) 42

	Score	Percentile
Outdoor	30	20
Mechanical	47	55
Computational	37	84
Scientific	27	12
Persuasive	46	66
Artistic	31	82
Literary	17	39
Musical	18	80
Social Service	29	15
Clerical	59	84

Case Study of Pulmonary Condition

Revised Minnesota Paper Form Board

Total Score: 35 Percentile Rank: 49 Table IV - 2

Occupational Interest Inventory – Advanced

	Score	Percentile
1. Pers. – Soc.	17	30
2. Nat.	13	30
3. Mech.	21	60
4. Bus.	29	80
5. Ar.	11	1
6. Sci.	29	90
7. Verbal	16	50
8. Manip.	16	50
9. Comp.	23	90

With regard to vocational interests, Mr. Jones, from the beginning of his evaluation, stated that he did not care what kind of work he did so long as it got him out of the house. The staff found that Mr. Jones required less frequent usage of his oxygen supply when he felt at ease in a given situation. He did express concern and fear over his physical status. It was the recommendation of the Center staff that client enter the workshop for a three-month period with reevaluation after one month in order to further evaluate his tolerance and to allow for work hardening.

During this time the Division of Vocational Rehabilitation counselor was to explore possible employment near his home. The client had, during the evaluation, shown progress in his determination and attitude toward employment. Findings and recommendations of the center were discussed with the client, and he was in agreement toward continued workshop experience. Mr. Jones' work tolerance had increased up to five plus hours a day, but he still required usage of oxygen supply about thirty seconds out of a thirty-minute period. This was actually not as much as the client thought he would require. The psychological component surrounding his reaction to his disease was clearly demonstrated.

Because of the increase in tolerance, the counselor discussed the case with the Social Security Trust Fund Counselor who agreed to take over the case using Trust Funds for extended evaluation. A counseling session was held with the client about transfer to a new counselor to insure that no feelings of rejection were allowed to form and to turn the transfer into a positive step. Further discussions were held with the client and Trust Fund counselor regarding his performance during evaluation. Interests fell into computational and clerical areas, but aptitudes, as can be seen in the previously given findings, were generally below average in both time and quality. They were average and somewhat better in basic math areas. Overall performance, as seen in bench samples, was up to standards, except for keeping up the pace. Manual dexterity as tested was found to be very poor, even for his dominant hand. When two-handed operations were required, he fell into the fifteenth percentile. It was therefore felt that if selective placement for this gentleman was to be carried out outside of an actual sheltered workshop or home setting, it would have to be non-factory because of pollutants, near home because of transportation, sedentary and environmentally and socially adaptative to use of oxygen supply. This left very few placement prospects available.

Consultation with the District Medical Consultant surrounding medical status of the client during evaluation showed that the client still required portable oxygen equipment but that he could tolerate five to six hours sedentary employment per day. The follow-up pulmonary function studies carried out during this evaluation period showed, in comparison to his previous testing, minimal deterioration in all parameters.

The counselor, during the period from March to May, continued to see the client in a supportive counseling manner on a weekly to biweekly basis. The counseling dealt with his depression about not being able to obtain employment, his medical condition and financial status.

On April 7, 1972, the counselor had contact with the client's physician at the Rehabilitation Hospital as well as other hospital personnel regarding the possibility of employment for his client as a utility aide where he would clean and sterilize packaging equipment (no problem with his oxygen supply), do filing, photocopying and minor record keeping. It was felt, after thorough discussion, however, that Mr. Jones would not benefit from employment in that hospital because it might tend to increase his dependency on that facility.

The counselor made contact with various employers near the client's home during the first two weeks of April, but no employer would take the chance on someone who required the use of the oxygen supply. Various reasons given for not even interviewing the client, aside from no openings, were insurance risk, chance of an attack and customer nonacceptance.

One company which ran a catalogue showroom did however express interest in Mr. Jones. Based upon the counselor's discussion with the manager, an appointment was scheduled for April 15, 1972. The job involved was clearly within his capacities: the taking of phone orders and on occasion, some personal contact. All the required recordkeeping was within his capacity.

Mr. Jones was interviewed on the 15th. It was understood that the job opening would still have to be cleared with the main office and that manager would have to discuss the oxygen unit with the office staff. It was left that they would contact Mr. Jones or the counselor. On April 21st, the manager of the company called the counselor to notify him that no opening existed for Mr. Jones. She was very sorry and she would have liked to help, but the company decided not to fill the job. The counselor saw the client at the Center and informed him of this decision. Mr. Jones' attendance at the Center during the past month had become sporadic because of transportation problems. His son was unable to take him everyday, and use of Center transportation could not be arranged.

On May 7, 1972, the counselor made a home visit to the client to discuss discontinuation of the client from workshop program at the Center. Mr. Jones had clearly shown that he had gained maximum benefit from the program, and transportation was still a major problem. The goal of showing Mr. Jones that he did have a work tolerance and was able to work five to six hours was accomplished. It was agreed that employment in sales or light clerical areas in a hospital or store would still be the best objective at this time.

It was felt that the question of reasonable expectation of benefit from Division of Vocational Rehabilitation services had been answered, and Mr. Jones was accepted for services. However, it was also felt that provision of vocational rehabilitation services would not result in a savings to the Social Security Trust Fund, and, therefore, he was removed from said program. Counselor did not transfer the case to a general caseload because it was felt that additional transferring of client would be detrimental to goals so far accomplished. The plan of action to help client continued to be counseling and guidance with continual job exploration. Convalescent hospitals near Mr. Jones' home were contacted, but no openings for someone with his limitations and lack of education existed.

During June, numerous contacts were made with a local hospital and its personnel department, pulmonary department and chief of pulmonary services (who happened to be client's physician) in an effort to develop a utility aide position for him in that department. Job duties would be similar to those explored at the Rehabilitation Hospital. Over the next three months, negotiations were held with the hospital, but no progress was made because of an overall job freeze.

The client was placed in contact with the State Employment Service during this month for additional help in selective placement. As a result of this, the Division of Vocational Rehabilitation counselor met with an employer who required someone to answer his company's telephone. An interview for the client was arranged. The employer needed a part-time clerk six hours per day for this position. The client met with the employer on August 7th and was hired at $2.25 per hour to start the following week.

Followup by the counselor on August 17th found that Mr. Jones was being terminated from the job at the end of the week because the employer was taking back an employee who had worked there previously and who was able to do more than Mr. Jones. The client was advised to maintain contact with the employment service. The counselor would also continue to see him and seek employment for him. When the client was seen in September, the counselor discussed the possibilities of a job at his home, monitoring fire calls using short-wave radios and tape recordings. This position was developed through community contacts established by the counselor. Mr. Jones, if hired, would work as a sub-contractor earning $25.00 per week. This would help meet his medical needs. The job required phoning an insurance adjuster seven days a week, two times daily. The advantages of this type of job were discussed with client. There were no transportation problems and if he had another attack or set-back, someone else in the family could cover the job for him. He would also be able to do this without pressure and at his own pace. Also the factor of weather did not come into play. The job's major drawback was that it did not remove him from the home.

On October 15, 1972, Mr. Jones started the job. This occurred after a month and one-half during which he was interviewed and the equipment ordered and installed. Counseling during this period focussed on his fears of not getting the job. These fears were caused by the contractor's representative being on vacation as well as in getting equipment installed.

The client's case was closed, "employed, sheltered work," on December 20, 1972.

RETROSPECT:

This client prior to onset of illness, could have been classified as a semi-skilled worker with limited education and skill, prerequisite to learning more advanced technical material. These factors would prevent advancement into more technical areas requiring advanced training.

We did not have any information regarding his premorbid personality which might have been helpful in better understanding his depression.

Superimposing upon his prior employment limitations, he had the additional factors imposed by his illness which further restricted his employability. Environmental factors clearly had to be considered (such as dust and weather conditions). Both his need for and his psychological dependency upon a portable oxygen supply were further problems to employment. Mr. Jones' depression superimposed on top of his severe pulmonary problems imposed other restrictions. In the realm of transporatation, many problem areas existed. No public transportation was present where he lived and he was unable to drive because of a lack of insurance and more important, by fear of an attack while driving. The family car was needed by his wife in order to get to her job which supported the family, making him dependent upon his children for transportation. Vocationally, his medical restrictions requiring sedentary employment when taken in conjunction with his education, acted as further limitations to employment. One can clearly see the numerous strikes against Mr. Jones in trying to reassume his role as head of the household.

Critical to the placement of any severely restricted pulmonary client is employer and community acceptance — one can go on at length regarding this critical area but it is not felt necessary to delve into this in a case study.

One final question to be pondered was whether early psychological treatment would not have substantially reduced the client's fears and concerns over his illness and related problems.

The client's continual need for medication and ongoing medical treatment, as well as probable rehospitalization, must always be taken into consideration in defining a vocational goal for a pulmonary case.

At the writing of this report, the client has again been hospitalized in a Rehabilitation Hospital for chronic obstructive pulmonary disease, chronic bronchitis and emphysema. This is his fourth admission to that hospital since 1971. Unlike his previous admissions, Mr. Jones can now return to a job which is being maintained by his family while he is hospitalized. The job duties consist of monitoring fire calls using short wave radio and tape recorders in his home: a highly selective, sheltered, environmentally protected position.

DISCUSSION QUESTIONS

1. What types of jobs should be avoided by the person with pulmonary difficulties?
2. Under pulmonary disability, discuss the particular diagnostic information needed in rehabilitation work.
3. Discuss special needs for follow-along services for pulmonary disability cases (this is generally a deteriorating condition which stabilizes but does not heal).

SUGGESTED READING

Acciavatti, Richard E. Factors related to hospital readmission of tuberculosis patients. Ann Arbor Michigan, University Microfilms, 1962.

Cohen, Burton M. Therapeutic opportunities in chronic ventilatory disease. J Appl Therapeutics, 1966, 8:340-345.

Cohen, Burton M. Clinical estimation of breathlessness. J Med Soc N J, 1964, 61:23-26.

Hardy, Richard E. and Cull, John G. Severe Disabilities: Social and Rehabilitation Approaches. Springfield, Thomas, 1973

National Tuberculosis and Respiratory Disease Association. Introduction to respiratory disease. New York NTRDA, 1969.

National Tuberculosis and Respiratory Disease Association. Facts about selected respiratory conditions in the United States: Epidemiology and statistics division. New York, NTRDA, 1969.

National Tuberculosis and Respiratory Disease Association. Standards for tuberculosis treatment in the 1970's: A statement by the Ad Hoc committee on quality care for tuberculosis. New York, NTRDA, 1970.

National Tuberculosis and Respiratory Disease Association. Tuberculosis facts in the United States. New York, NTRDA, 1972.

Chapter 5

CASE STUDY OF CARDIOVASCULAR DISEASE

Discussion Questions
Suggested Reading

THE client, Mr. Fractus, first came to the attention of the Division of Vocational Rehabilitation when he was referred by the local office of the State Employment Service.

He was a 60-year old, married, caucasian male with twelve children, nine of them still living at home. They ranged in age from four to twenty-one. The client's wife was 44-years-old and a full-time housewife.

The family had recently arrived in the area from another state, as the client had a job as salesman with a petroleum company and was given this territory. The client was working parttime because of his cardiac disability.

Mr. Fractus' education was limited to two years of high school, however, he had served a carpenters apprenticeship and worked as a master carpenter for 35 years. The client served in the United States Army Medical Corp from 1925 to 1927 and was honorably discharged.

He had a driver's license and did drive although it was very tiring for him. Aside from what the client made when he was able to sell petroleum, his only income was $270 per month from Social Security Disability Benefits.

Upon questioning, the client stated he had recently been evaluated by the local Heart Association Evaluation Unit and had contact with the Division of Vocational Rehabilitation in the state he had come from. Further questioning brought out the fact that the client had owned a farm and worked very hard to support his large family. The client was a proud man who wanted to make it on his own and had only come for our services when he could not do it alone.

Before the client left the office, the counselor made sure that he had taken advantage of the Title 19 medical program and the Food Stamp program. Mr. Fractus was also informed of the local agencies and programs that might be of value to him while he waited for our evaluation to be completed, which normally took from two weeks to a month. A general medical examination was not arranged for the client at this time because of his very recent hospitalization and cardiac review. The case was now placed in Status 02, the client having signed all the forms required for our services.

Medical releases were sent out and a request for Social Security verification was made. Within two weeks data started to arrive.

1. Medical reports included a recent complete work-up by a cardiologist with EKG and x-ray of chest with barium swallow. The summary from all the medical reports indicated that the client had a hypertensive and arteriosclerotic cardiovascular disease, probable old myocardial infarction, myocardial fibrosis, coronary sclerosis and angina pectoris. His functional and therapeutic classification would be III-C.

2. Psychological reports received indicated that Mr. Fractus was a very verbal, forcefully engaging gentleman (now a salesman) who readily discussed recent complaints. He described becoming readily fatigued, so that he could work only two or three days a week. He mentioned poor circulation and blackouts.

In summary, Mr. Fractus appeared to be a gentleman who had been self-sufficient for many years. He was now reacting with some bitterness to changes in occupation and a much lowered income as he tried to maintain his self-esteem. He was somewhat ambivalent but seemed willing to settle for some financial aid (though it meant dependency) if his physical condition warranted it.

3. Social summary received reviewed the family situation and stated that the client first became ill 5 years ago in 1968, was in and out of the hospital during 1969 and was forced to sell his farm before his condition stabilized enough to begin selling oil products. The client got into selling these products, as during his

recuperation, the company, which had been selling oil to him to run the machinery on his farm, offered to train him so he could sell their products. He took a four-week training program and was given a territory. He sold on commission and his income, after expenses, was very small. The client has been selling for a year.

By the middle of May, two and one-half weeks after the client was first seen, there was sufficient material for review by our medical consultant. We were fortunate, in this particular case, that our consultant was a cardiologist. After reviewing the medical material, he felt the client could work or be trained for some sedentary operation. However, the number of hours the client could work and other limitations imposed could best be discovered in a work trial situation.

The client was contacted and arrangements were made for him to be reviewed at the local sheltered workshop. He showed an interest in furniture refinishing, which fitted in well with what was being done at the workshop.

A month after the referral, sufficient documentation had been received so that we could accept this client, based on the fact that he had a hypertensive, arteriosclerotic, cardiovascular disease that made it impossible for him to work as a farmer or carpenter, his former occupations. Because of the disability, he was having trouble stabilizing himself in the sales work. However he did have rehabilitation potential because the medical review indicated he could work in some sedentary job. The case was placed in Status 10.

Before the workshop evaluation was completed, the client came into the office to inform the counselor that he did not want to stay at the workshop. He had received a new offer from the oil company, which meant they were going to pay some of his expenses, and he now felt he may have a better opportunity of developing this job into a profitable venture. He was feeling better and had clearance from his local doctor. The counselor had been in contact with client's local physician, and we agreed that client should try this new opportunity. The following plan was written and the client was placed in Status 14 (Counseling and Guidance Only).

Vocational Objective: Salesman

The client has a hypertensive, arteriosclerotic, cardiovascular disease with an old myocardial fibrosis, coronary sclerosis and angina pectoris and possible hyperventilation syndrome. Review of the Heart Association Work Evaluation Unit indicated the client could do sedentary work which did not involve great exertion. The client indicated he was interested in a selling job and had contact with an oil company with the idea that he would sell oil to garages on a wholesale basis. Since the client seemed interested in this kind of work, the counselor felt this may be the best job for this man due to his many physical limitations. The counselor would assist the client with counseling and guidance while he tried to make a go of this business.

All went well for about four months, and the counselor was about to close the case when, on October 23, Mr. Fractus reappeared. He told the counselor that his oil selling job had become limited due to the fact that he had another mild heart attack and had not been able to work.

In counseling the client about this new problem, the counselor suggested another type of work, such as Fuller Brush selling on the phone or some sedentary job in a local factory. It was even suggested that maybe the client's wife should go to work and the client stay at home. The client was to think over the possibilities and let the counselor know.

Three months went by with no word from the client, so in January the counselor called the client and was informed by his wife that the client had just returned to selling oil.

The client seemed to be doing better, and again the counselor was ready to close the case when client finally admitted that he was really not able to drive all over selling oil and had not really been successful. After much counseling, the client was now able to accept some help in setting up a new vocational goal. Mr. Fractus still felt he would like to be in his own business. He based this on his experience with his farm and the need for working at his own rate, stopping when he felt pain or became tired. The counselor also felt that with his disability, personality and experience a home business might be the most practical objective. Another plus was the client's family, who could help him with the work.

The counselor realized that this client was well motivated and needed to do as much as possible himself, or he would lose his self-esteem. The counseling centered on what steps the client would need to take in exploring business ventures.

The first step was to arrange to have the client meet with the Small Business Administration. The counselor called their office and an appointment was set up for the client. It was explained to the client how this appointment could be used to start his search for what he thought would be a good business for his family and himself. He would review the franchises available with the Small Business Administration.

At the same interview the client had questions about his Social Security situation and the counselor called the local Social Security office so these could be answered. It is very common for clients who are on Social Security Disability Benefits to worry about losing them if they return to work. Since very often this is the only income that the client has, the thought of losing it can be a strong deterrent to his starting any work program. A complete and understanding discussion of the work incentives built into the program and how they can affect the client in his work plan can be very important to the success of his rehabilitation.

When the client was next seen, he had an idea of the type of business he felt he wanted. The client stated he had reviewed many different businesses and found that an auto-simonizing establishment could be most practical for him. He hoped that his wife and sons could do most of the heavy work and he would help parttime. Mr. Fractus also thought that he could sell the oil products at the same time, thus increasing his income.

The counselor discussed the idea at length with the client, and it was decided that the client would contact the franchise company and get all the information. He would also check with the local Chamber of Commerce to see if they thought a business of this type was practical in the community. The counselor pointed out to the client that contact with the Chamber could be important when and if he was ready to go into business.

After the client left, the counselor reviewed the information in the folder to be sure that no steps in the planning had been left out. Since the case was now a year old, the counselor decided that some updating of medical and psychological information was warranted before getting too much further into the business planning. This was especially important in this case as the client had had some minor cardiac arrests in the recent past.

It was now time for the counselor to play the "devil's advocate" and question all the details to make sure that the client was being practical in his evaluation of the business and its potential. All of the possible pitfalls were reviewed. As it turned out, the client had given much thought to most of them beforehand and was ready with logical and practical answers. He had even gone so far as to line up potential customers. The only fly in the ointment, and it was a big one, was at what location the business was to be conducted.

The Fractus' home is located in a suburban area. It is not on a thoroughfare and he does not have a garage. For the type of business that client had in mind it was necessary to have a central location near a busy road if the client was to get customers.

This problem looked insurmountable when initially discussed with the client. However, in a few days the client returned to say he had made arrangements to rent a local garage in the center of town at a very reasonable rate. Mr. Fractus said the building was all ready to go. He was waiting for a word as to the plan. Meanwhile, he would go to the city hall to find out about licenses, tax stamps, etc.

The counselor was impressed by the client's ingenuity in overcoming the problem and his foresight in checking some of the details. These actions tended to clear away the counselor's remaining doubts about the client's ability to succeed in the business.

The next step was for the counselor to contact the company that supplied the equipment for the business. The following letter was sent:

"Dear Mr. Smith:

A client of mine, Mr. Animi Fractus, has indicated to me an interest in getting into the business you represent. Since it is a function of the Division of Vocational Rehabilitation to help handicapped clients find employment, we may be interested in helping if it is feasible for him.

The client has a cardiac condition and so it will be necessary for us to know the amount of physical exertion necessary for doing this type of work. We understand he has a large family and would not do much of the actual polishing. His prime function would be to line up customers. However, he would have to be responsible for the business; so before we can consider helping finance this venture, I would appreciate knowing more about your company.

Since the client is interested in getting started in something, your prompt reply would be appreciated.

Very truly yours,"

While waiting for the reply to the letter, the client's physical condition was reviewed by his cardiologist and our medical consultant. They both agreed that client's physical condition was still classified as III-C. This classification is based on the American Heart Association's scale, which is divided into two areas; the functional classification covering an estimate of what the patient's heart will allow him to do and the therapeutic classification indicating the amount of physical activity which is advised.

Class III then refers to a patient with cardiac disease resulting in marked limitations of physical activity. This type of patient is comfortable at rest. Even less than ordinary physical activity causes fatigue, palpitation, dyspnea or anginal pain.

The "C" designation refers to patients with cardiac disease whose ordinary physical activity should be moderately restricted and whose more strenuous efforts should be discontinued. Using the above guide, we can see that the type of activity involved in the simonizing business was possible for our client.

Even though the client had a strong motivation, the counselor still had the responsibility of seeing if his intelligence level and personality would make this client suitable to run a customer contact business. Updated review by the psychologist showed that the client had a full scale I.Q. of 105 on the Weschler Adult Intelligence Scale. His verbal score was 103 and his performance score 108. He seemed to be a little above average in working with numbers. He had ability to do average clerical tasks, such as keeping records and arithmetical figuring. There were no counter-indications to his interacting with people. In fact, all the objective tests seemed to indicate he would succeed in a business.

The last variable to consider was the client's wife and family. Could they and would they be able to play their part in the business? The counselor interviewed the wife at length, discussed her health, her responsibilities at home with the children, her feelings about the business and her plans to assist. The counselor was happy to see that she was an intelligent woman who had been assisting her husband right along and had a good understanding of the responsibilities and disadvantages of a business. She had figured out a schedule for herself and the children so that there would be continuous help to do the heavier work in the business.

By the end of May, just one year after the case was referred, a plan was written for the auto-simonizing business. The company had contacted the counselor by phone and all the details worked out. The counselor had checked out the company and found them to be a reliable and reputable concern.

In writing the plan the medical problem was reviewed and the history and background were given. Then the counselor went on to say that client's prime responsibility would be to line up customers. He had already been able to do this with good success. Basically his wife and family will do most of the simonizing while he does the selling and customer contact. Based on the type of activity the client would do in the business and the good family back-up, the counselor felt the client should be assisted. Medical and psychological reports showed no counterindication to the client's success. The Small Business Administration had also been contacted and had offered advice.

The counselor would assist the client with the business through counseling and guidance during the setting-up and training period offered by the company. A grand opening would be arranged. The counselor would work with client until he was doing well and was stabilized.

The case was placed in Status 18 — training. While the client was learning to use the equipment, the counselor visited often to see how things were going. The client was learning quickly and even insisted upon simonizing the counselor's car. Sometimes a counselor has to make some personal sacrifices to expedite the rehabilitation of a client. This was one of those times, and counselor had his car simonized. It turned out very well and was proof positive that client was ready for his grand opening.

It was important to the future of the client's business to get as much publicity as possible. The Division of Vocational Rehabilitation and the company's public relations firm worked together to obtain as much as possible. The company was to be represented by the vice-president and other company dignitaries. We arranged to have the local political and business leaders available, as well as local and state press. Mr. Fractus had been prepared for all the exciting events to come so that the excitement would not cause any undue physical distress.

The grand opening was held, and as is common at these types of events, it rained as if the biblical flood was going to recur, but that did not dampen the feeling of optimism that the client had. The business was now in full operation and the case was placed in Status 22 (In Employment).

Two weeks later a problem developed, and a supplementary plan had to be written:

> The client's business was going along well but a problem had come up. Since he had only one machine, when it overheated or malfunctioned he was not able to do any work. This happened twice. The company did repair the machine without charge but it took time. Even when the machine worked well it would heat up after many cars and the company had recommended a supplemental machine to help prevent most of these problems. Since the client was on a limited income and with the expenses he had had, on his own, in starting the business he still needed our help to get the item so that his business could continue to progress.

This was the last problem and last plan necessary in getting Mr. Fractus started in his business. After one year and four months from first referral, counselor was able to close the case. The last contact note stated

> The client has now been in business for four months and the business seems to be doing quite well for a new business. He is stabilized and is slowly working up. He is presently making a profit of about $4.00 per week over and above all his many expenses. For a new business this is very good. The client works primarily as a salesman and contact man

while the family does most of the simonizing work. This fits well with client's disability.

EPILOGUE

It would be nice to say the client had no more problems and, as far as the success of the business went, he did not. His profit kept increasing and he made many new customers. Since he was severely disabled, his Social Security continued to carry him over the initial financial problems inherent in a new business.

Mr. Fractus has his case reopened about one-and-one-half years later when his hearing and eyes started to cause problems. He was evaluated and received a hearing aid and glasses. The case was again closed; the client is working successfully as a salesman in the family business and this case was closed as rehabilitated. Form SS-853 was forwarded to Baltimore.

OPINION AND EVALUATION

This case is an example of a man who had to go from a very active life to almost a completely sedentary one. The activity he was used to had come through physical action; now it had to come through intellectual action. The business was the intellectual action that was needed by the client to help him adjust to his disability and not lose his self-respect in his own eyes or those of his family.

The family also gained from being involved in the business. The children felt they were important in helping their parents. Since the busiest season was during the summer months, the children were able to continue in school. Mrs. Fractus took care of the records and was available to her children and her husband. She could keep an eye on him so that he did not over exert and yet the client did not feel that he was being supported by his wife. By continuing in their normal roles, the effect of the disability on the internal family structure was minimized. Problems that do develop in the marriage when the husband becomes incapacitated did not occur.

Without a real purpose in life, this man would have developed many emotional problems and the family would have disintegrated. The counselor felt this would have occurred if another year or two had gone by without any change in the client's life style. The client's losing contact with us for a few periods of time early in the case was evidence of his feeling of hopelessness and despair. If close followup had not been made by the counselor, then this would have been another lost soul, a case closed because of no contact, and a man with much to offer to his family and himself would have been wasted.

DISCUSSION QUESTIONS

1. Discuss the special diagnostic information needed in rehabilitation work with cardiovascular disease victims.
2. Discuss work to be avoided by this disability group.
3. Discuss the "cardiac personality".
4. Discuss the vocational implications of cardiovascular accident.

SUGGESTED READING

Acker, J.E. Role of the cardiac work evaluation units in cardiac rehabilitation. In Rehabilitation in Cardiac Disease. Boston Tufts University, School of Medicine, 1967.

Bakker, C.B. Psychological factors in angina pectoris. Psychosomatics, 8(1):43, 1967.

Bakker, C.B. and Levenson, R.M. Determinants of angina pectoris. Psychosom Med 29(6):621, 1967.

Bellak, L. and Haselkorn, F. Psychological aspects of cardiac illness and rehabilitation. Soc Casework, 37:483, 1956.

Brandaleone, H. Driving and the coronary patient. J Rehabil, 32(2):97, 1966.

Chambers, W. and Reiser, M.F. Emotional stress in the precipitation of congestive heart failure. Psychosom, 15:38, 1953.

Cleveland, S.E. and Johnson, D.L. Personality patterns in young males with coronary disease. Psychosom Med, 24(6):600, 1962.

Cook, W.L. Suggestions in cardiac rehabilitation. In Rehabilitation in Cardiac Disease. Boston, Tufts University, School of Medicine, 1967.

DeWolf, A., Barrell, R., and Cummings, J. Patient variables in emotional response to hospitalization for physical illness. J Consult Psychol, 30:68, 1966.

Dudley, D.L., Martin, C.J., and Holmes, T.H. Dyspnea: Psychologic and physiologic observations. J Psychosom Res, 11(4):325, 1968.

Fisher, S.H. The cardiac homemaker. J Rehabil, 32(2):74, 1966.
Fox, H.M., Rizzo, N.D., and Sanford, G. Psychological observations of patients undergoing mitral surgery: A study of stress. Psychosom Med, 16(3):186, 1954.
Gardberg, M. Remarks on the rehabilitation of the cardiac patient. J La Med Soc, 109:335, 1957.
Gelfand, D. Factors related to unsuccessful vocational adjustment of cardiac patients. In Rehabilitation in Cardiac Disease. Boston Tufts University, School of Medicine, 1967.
Gelfand, D. Experience at the cardiac classification unit, Southeastern Pennsylvania. In Rosenbaum, F.F. and Belknap, E.L. (Eds.) Work and the Heart. New York, P.B. Hoeber, Inc., 1959.
Geldea, E.F. Special features of personality which are common to certain psychosomatic disorders. Psychosom Med, 11:273, 1949.
Ginsparg, S.L. and Satten, J. Psychiatric aspects of rehabilitation in coronary artery illness. Proceedings of the American Psychological Annual Convention, 1970.
Goldwater, L.J. and Bronstein, L.H. Fifteen years of cardiac work classification (etiology of heart disease in relation to employment). J Occup Med, 1:145, 1959.
Gray, R.M., Reinhardt, A.M., and Ward, J.R. Psychosocial factors involved in the rehabilitation of persons with cardiovascular diseases. Rehabil Lit, 30:354, 1969.
Hagan, J. Vocational counseling in heart disease. J Rehabil, 32(2):62, 1966.
Hardy, R.E. and Cull, J.G. Severe disabilities: Social and Rehabilitation Approaches. Springfield, Thomas, 1973.
Heath, M.J. Myocardial infarction – A personal account. J Rehabil, 32(2):46, 1966.
Hellerstein, H.K. Active physical reconditioning of coronary patients. In Rehabilitation in Cardiac Disease. Boston Tufts University, School of Medicine, 1967.
Hellerstein, H.K. and Ford, A.B. Rehabilitation of the cardiac patients. JAMA, Vol. 164-225, 1957.
Hellerstein, H.K. and Hornsten, T.R. Assessing and preparing the patient for return to a meaningful, productive life. J Rehabil, 32(2):48, 1966.
Hurst, J.W. and Logue, R.B. The Heart Arteries and Veins. New York McGraw-Hill Book Company, 1966.
Kaplan, S. Psychological aspects of cardiac disease: A study of patients experiencing mitral commissurotomy. Psychosom Med, 18:221, 1956.
Katz, L.N. Psychological aspects of heart disease. Psychosom Med, 26:413, 1964.
Lebovits, B.A., Shekelle, R.B., Ostfeld, A.M., and Paul, O. Prospective and retrospective psychological studies of coronary heart disease. Psychosom Med, 29(3):265, 1967.

Margolis, D. Resource material to aid in prevention and treatment. J Rehabil, 32(2):101, 1966.
Mordkoff, A.M. and Parsons, O.A. The coronary personality: A critique. Psychosom Med, 29(1):1, 1967.
Morris, W.H.M. The coronary farmer, J Rehabil, 32(2):76, 1966.
Morris, W.H.M. Heart disease in the farmer, In Rehabilitation in Cardiac Disease. Boston, Tufts University, School of Medicine, 1967.
Nolan, J.C. Vocational assessment. J Rehabil, 32(2):61, 1966.
Pohlmann, K.E. Labor and the coronary worker. J Rehabil, 32(2):79, 1966.
Rasof, B., Linde, L.M., and Dunn, O.J. Intellectual development in children with congenital heart disease. Child Dev, 38(4):1043, 1967.
Sparkman, D.R. Place of vocational rehabilitation administration in cardiac rehabilitation. In Rehabilitation in Cardiac Disease. Boston Tufts University, School of Medicine, 1967.
Thornton, John. Waiver statute, second injury laws and other compensation law devices as related to rehabilitation. In Rehabilitation in Cardiac Disease. Boston Tufts University, School of Medicine, 1967.
Verwoerdt, A. and Dovenmuehle, R. Heart disease and depression. Geriatrics, 18:856, 1964.
Weaver, N.K. Industry and the coronary worker. J Rehabil, 32(2):77, 1966.
Weaver, N.K. Selective placement of the cardiac in industry. In Rehabilitation of Cardiac Disease. Boston, Tufts University, School of Medicine, 1967.
White, J. and Sweet, W. Pain, Its Mechanism and Neurosurgical Control. Springfield, Thomas, 1955.
Whitehouse, F.A. "Cardiacs" without heart disease. J Rehabil, 33:56, 1967.
Whitehouse, F.A. The cardiac work evaluation unit as a specialized team approach. J Rehabil, 32(2):66, 1966.
Wright, B.A. Physical Disability – A Psychological Approach. New York, Harper & Row, 1960.

Chapter 6

MENTAL RETARDATION

>Case Number One
>Case Number Two
>Case Number Three
>Case Number Four
>Summary
>Discussion Questions
>Suggested Reading

MENTAL retardation is a very broad concept. Terms that have been used to describe this condition have been idiot, moron, imbecile and feeble-minded.

The variation in the terms and the method of handling the problems of these individuals in the past present a challenge to those interested in the possibility of helping parents and these individuals themselves make necessary adjustment.

Currently, the terminology used is mildly retarded, moderately retarded, severely retarded and profoundly retarded. In some school systems there are classes for the mildly and moderately retarded. The other two groups are left to be provided for by the parents, through private schools or through institutionalization in state homes and training schools.

In 1943 the national Vocational Rehabilitation Act was expanded to include the mentally retarded who met the eligibility requirements. These requirements were:
1. A physical or mental disability with limitations.
2. The disability must create a substantial barrier to employment.
3. There must be a reasonable expectation that the individual will be capable of being employed after the service is rendered.

In order to determine whether the individual met the requirements, a general medical examination and a psychological examination were secured to determine the intellectual level. Usually this was the result of an intelligence test. Those individuals in the mildly retarded group usually were accepted for rehabilitation services, and some of the moderately retarded, but most generally the two lower groups were not found to meet the third requirement.

Special education classes for the higher levels were established in many of the schools throughout the nation. Generally the classes started in the elementary school, but as time went by the students reached the secondary schools. They were going to the high school classes, but many of the parents were not satisfied with the program available to their children. Educators who were not happy with the situation, also, began to seek other ways to meet the needs of these students. Out of this searching, there developed what was termed the work-study program in the high school. This is a program in which the student goes to school for one-half of the day and then works on a trial basis, in industry or in a workshop setting, for the other half of the day. The teacher usually is freed to work with the employers and community for part of the day, so that the work experience will be relevant to the classroom and so the employers will gain more understanding of the capabilities of the mentally retarded. This is usually a cooperative venture, with the local school district, the state Department of Education, the Vocational Education Program and the state Rehabilitation Program.

Many private agencies have developed special training and workshop programs for the mentally retarded. Some of the workshop programs have been developed for the more severely retarded. The intention of the workshop is to train the individual so he will be capable of working and earning some of the expenses toward his living. The individual will at least be busy and not just sitting watching television, or doing nothing during the day. These workshops generally try to secure subcontract work. The work may consist of packaging, assemblying or some similar process. This activity enables the private workshop to train some individuals who may go into competitive employment after finishing the training. Others can be employed at the workshop in a sheltered environment.

The regulations of the rehabilitation program were expanded in 1968 to allow for extended periods of evaluation to determine vocational potential. This allows for a performance evaluation in order to help the counselor determine if the individual meets the third eligibility requirement. This performance evaluation is usually secured from one of the workshops in the region. This procedure enables the counselor to develop much greater knowledge of the ability of the client.

In terms of the rehabilitation program and the factors which enable the program to be successful with some of the mentally retarded, many variables have been found to play an important part. The adjustment of the home from which the individual comes is a very important factor. The satisfaction which the individual attains from being in a work setting may be considerably eroded by the critical views of a father or a mother expressed to the child.

Another important factor is the way in which the community has treated the individual. If he has been unable to participate in any of the activities of his own age, it will probably require some special training to overcome the hesitancy which he and his parents may feel. There may be an overprotectiveness on the part of the family. In working in this area, the counselor will need to carefully assess the total situation before the plan is finally completed. The family must be carefully considered in the development of the plan for the mentally retarded.

Rehabilitation services are becoming more accessible to the mentally retarded. Federal government jobs have been opened to the retarded on a performance evaluation instead of the written test. Some states have developed the same criteria in order to help the mentally retarded into suitable jobs. Many of the retarded will do the work with which the more able workers become bored because of the monotony of it.

In order to be placed on a job tryout with the federal or state governments, usually the rehabilitation counselor must certify that the individual is physically capable of doing the work, that the individual should be capable of doing the work from the mental ability level, that he is capable of managing his free time and that he can accept responsibility for getting to and from the job. In order to certify to these requirements, the counselor must know the client that he is servicing.

In working in the field of the mentally retarded, it must be recognized that emotional problems are in many instances a part of the problem with which we are dealing. The program must have the capability of working with these problems in order to provide the special help some of these individuals may require. The use of mental health clinics, the services of a psychiatrist, psychologist and other professional workers will sometimes be needed in the rehabilitation process.

The importance of the rehabilitation methodology of working with each person or client on a one-to-one basis is very essential in this program. Each client is considered as an important person, with special interests, personality and capabilities. A plan is designed with that person, especially, to meet his vocational potential. The plan is one in which the individual has had an active part in formulating. To explain the way in which a counselor may work with a client who is mentally retarded, some case histories are included.

CASE NUMBER ONE

JOE VINER
Referred by high school teacher.
Disability: Primary, mental retardation; secondary, cerebral palsy, involving muscular coordination, speech and gait.
Age: 17 years.
Joe is in high school, in a special education class. He was referred because his teacher thought he would be a good candidate for the work-study program.
Family: Father and mother, one older sister and a younger brother, both apparently normal. Father drives a truck for a local concern. Mother is in the home. Both mother and father graduated from high school. The older sister was apparently a very good student and earned a scholarship when she graduated from high school. Is now attending a state college, nearby. The younger brother is in the seventh grade. No apparent problems with his school work.

Family income is not great, but it does appear to be adequate as the family is buying their home. It is a small, modest home, neat and clean. Joe and his younger brother share a bedroom. They appear to be well adjusted to each other and get along well together. There was a problem with the sister the last two years in high school. The mother stated that she believed the daughter did not know quite how to explain Joe's condition to her high school friends. His awkwardness, his speech difficulty and the accompanying drooling embarrassed his sister. The mother stated the relationship had improved considerably since the daughter has gone away to school.

Joe has many friends in school and they appear to accept him. He goes to all high school activities and is a strong supporter of school functions.

There is warm acceptance of Joe by both his parents. His father occasionally has taken time off from work in the spring and summer and has taken both of the boys fishing.

Joe writes poorly and is difficult to understand when he speaks. Both of these factors have influenced his school work.

The psychological examination indicated that Joe was in the mildly retarded group. A full scale I.Q. score of 63 was obtained on the Weschler Scale.

Interested in mechanical fields.

Medical diagnosis was congenital cerebral palsy with neuromuscular involvement and speech difficulty.

Father and mother accompanied Joe to the initial interview with the rehabilitation counselor. They explained that the special education work-study program had been discussed by the special education teacher. They were concerned about Joe's future and so wished to know about the rehabilitation program. The counselor explained the program, how a plan is developed for each individual, the services that might be provided, etc.

A survey was taken and the parents gave permission to secure the psychological and medical information.

The work-study program was outlined in detail. The father suggested a small, all-purpose mechanical repair shop that might be interested in cooperating with the work-study program.

The first year Joe worked in three different establishments. He worked in a restaurant as a bus boy and did not particularly like this work. His second job was in the small mechanical repair business which his father mentioned. He liked this work and the people liked him. Here he functioned as a helper and errand boy.

The third experience of his first year was in a sheltered workshop. He was on an assembly production line. He enjoyed working with the people in the workshop but did not like the work as well as the work in the repair shop.

During the vacation between spring and fall, Joe was able to work full-time in the repair shop. When school started again in the fall, the plan was developed to allow Joe to work there on the work-study program, part-time the first semester and then to go to work full-time in the shop in the final semester. He will get credit for this work-study and will attend terminating ceremonies with his class. If everything goes as planned and Joe continues to do good work in the repair shop, he will have a full-time job there after his school program is completed.

Joe's parents have been closely involved in this plan, and although they realize there will be problems with Joe in reference to marriage, etc., they are of the opinion that this is a very good plan for him. He is still in the work study program in the first semester of his last year.

CASE NUMBER TWO

ROWENA VITALIE

Referred by an interviewer in the State Employment Service. She was referred because of her inability to hold a job. Rowena was a high school graduate. She had completed high school when she was nineteen years old.

Age: 21 years.

Family: Rowena is the only child of Mr. and Mrs. Vitalie. Italian descent. Her father is a machinist in a local manufacturing plant. They own their home on the west side.

Mrs. Vitalie accompanied Rowena to the initial interview. She appears to be very concerned about her daughter and said that both parents did not know what to do about the problem Rowena has of securing and holding a job. The rehabilitation program was explained to Mrs. Vitalie and Rowena. The requirement that there must be a physical or mental disability was discussed. Mrs. Vitalie said before they would go even so far as to have a medical examination, she wanted to discuss this with Mr. Vitalie. The counselor agreed this would be fine because it was not evident to the observer that there was any kind of qualifying disability. Mrs. Vitalie thanked the counselor and said she would phone him and inform him as to their decision.

Mrs. Vitalie was a small, dark woman, neatly dressed. Rowena was taller than her mother, neatly and attractively dressed. She was a pretty girl.

Two days later the counselor received a phone call from Mrs. Vitalie stating they would like to have the medical examination to determine whether there was a physical disability. Rowena would come to the office to make the arrangements. An appointment was made for a general medical examination with their family doctor.

The employment interviewer who had referred Rowena was phoned to see if a GATB test had been done for Rowena. There were test results available, he informed the counselor, and he would forward a copy to the office of the counselor.

The medical report received and all findings were normal, no physical disability.

GATB results were received and were found to be very low, no pattern.

Both GATB results and medical reports were discussed by the counselor and the medical consultant. It was the conclusion that a psychological evaluation should be secured. Mrs. Vitalie was phoned and asked if she and Rowena could come in for an interview. The appointment was made. They came in and the findings were discussed. The recommendation for a psychological test was made. At first Mrs. Vitalie was against having this as she thought this indicated that the counselor believed Rowena was "crazy" and she knew this wasn't so. After considerable explanation, it was agreed they would try this one more step for Rowena.

An evaluation was scheduled at an adult vocational school for a complete battery of tests.

The report was received and the results indicated that Rowena was functioning as a mildly retarded individual. Full scale I.Q. score on the Wechsler was 58. There were some indications of emotional problems present. The psychologist discussed the question of high school graduation. He pointed out that Rowena was a pretty girl, that her parents dressed her very attractively and that in the large high school where she attended, the classes were large and probably by just going to class and creating no problems, she was able to graduate. He indicated that although she was in the classes, she had no really close friends and she was unhappy because she really had no "boy friends."

On the basis of the psychological report, Rowena was accepted for the rehabilitation program as a mentally retarded client.

Mrs. Vitalie and Rowena came into the office to discuss the

development of a plan. The test results were interpreted to Mrs. Vitalie and she said they had thought something was wrong because Rowena wanted a job but had been unable to hold any she could find for more than a few days. These jobs had consisted of a sales clerk in a five and ten cent store, a counter waitress in a short-order restaurant and a job in a floral shop. She had been discharged from all of them.

The decision was made to have Rowena go to a sheltered workshop for several months to secure a performance evaluation for her. Plans were worked out for this evaluation. In approximately two weeks Rowena would start attending the workshop. All expenses except the tuition would be paid by Mr. and Mrs. Vitalie.

At the conclusion of the evaluation period it was determined that Rowena had good manual dexterity and that perhaps some type of assembly work would be suitable. A job was located in a fishing lure manufacturing plant and Rowena was placed in this job.

The rehabilitation counselor checked on her progress over a period of several months and Rowena appeared to be making a very good adjustment and the company was satisfied with her as a worker. Mr. and Mrs. Vitalie also came into the office to express their appreciation for services rendered to Rowena. The counselor "closed" the case.

Four months later Mrs. Vitalie phoned to make an appointment to see the counselor. She was upset because Rowena had made friends with a man approximately fifteen or twenty years older than she, and both Mr. and Mrs. Vitalie were opposed to this situation. She explained that this man and Rowena were planning to be married. The man worked somewhere close to the manufacturing plant where Rowena worked. The man was not a Catholic and the Vitalies were; however, he and Rowena were planning to be married in a civil ceremony. The counselor tried to point out that maybe things would work out all right for Rowena, but Mrs. Vitalie was not convinced when she left the office.

Approximately three months later Mrs. Vitalie made an appointment to see the counselor again. This time she came in and brought Rowena with her. Rowena had been married and had quit her job to keep house. After about six weeks of marriage the husband just left the home saying he couldn't stand Rowena any longer. In the discussion it was brought out that there had been dissension between Rowena and her husband almost from the very start of their marriage.

The counselor said he would visit the plant where Rowena had been employed and see if he could get the company to take her back. This was agreed upon. Rowena was to move back home and live with her parents. The counselor contacted the personnel man at the plant and it was agreed that Rowena was to go back to the same job she had before.

Follow-up contacts were made by the counselor and Rowena is now doing very well at the plant and the home situation appears to be pretty well adjusted once more.

This case indicates the need which is present in many cases of mental retardation. The importance of a "follow-along" service to provide for needed services, such as counseling, etc., does not stop when a job is secured. There is a need to have an opportunity to see a counselor when additional problems are encountered by the client.

CASE NUMBER THREE

ENRIQUE ALAVAREZ
Referred by Occupational Adjustment Service of Adult Vocational School. School dropout from a junior high school.
Age: 23 years and single.
Family: Mother on ADC; Father's whereabouts unknown.
Two brothers older and three sisters younger than Enrique in the home.
The occupational adjustment referred him because they were unable to find him any kind of work.
The counselor observed his behavior in the interview, and although Enrique said he had no disability of any kind, it was decided to secure the medical and psychological to find out about his situation.

Medical report indicated underweight, but no other physical findings.

The psychological report indicated a moderately retarded individual. Full scale Wechsler I.Q. score was 52.

As a result of this finding, a plan was made to send him to a sheltered workshop for a performance evaluation and perhaps for sheltered employment, if such was indicated. A workshop was contacted and a starting date agreed upon. This was discussed and explained to Enrique and it was apparently all settled.

Before the plan was placed in operation however, Enrique was caught burglarizing a grocery store one night. At the trial a plea was made for a probation period to allow Enrique to go into the rehabilitation program, but the probation was denied and Enrique is now serving a term in the state penitentiary. When he is discharged, it will be that much more difficult to develop a suitable plan for his rehabilitation.

CASE NUMBER FOUR

WILLIAM TARKEY

Re-referred by another rehabilitation client because he "needs help."
Age: 43 years and single.
Lives at 2301 Alada Way in a boarding house for welfare recipients

As he was a former rehabilitation client, the counselor indicated he would secure the record and see what the situation was. The applicant said he knew he could work if someone would give him a chance. He said that he had never learned to read but that he had learned to write his name. He is, and has been for a number of years, drawing welfare help as an AND case. He works part time for part of his room and board as a night watchman at the boarding house. He works from 11:00 p.m. until 5:00 a.m. He may sleep during this time but is there in case the phone rings or someone comes to the door.

William's nickname is "Big Bill." He is six feet, two inches tall and looks very thin.

It was agreed that the counselor would secure the record and then call the applicant in to go over the record with him.

The applicant's record was secured. The case had been known to the agency for over four years. A performance evaluation had been secured from a local workshop to determine his vocational potential. The report indicated that the client had been determined to have very little, if any, potential for employment, even in a sheltered situation. The rehabilitation counselor had helped him get on the welfare rolls. Physically, he was marked normal, except for the fact that he was underweight. He had been rejected for military service because he was illiterate.

"Big Bill" was called in for an interview and his friend, the other rehabilitation client, came in with him. During the interview, the applicant related a very recent experience he had gone through in trying to go from one particular address in the city to another. He stated he got lost and finally had to ask someone where he was and how he would get back to the boarding house. He said he was afraid to get on a bus, so he walked a considerable number of miles to get home.

The discussion centered on how well "Big Bill" was getting along on his welfare and the fact that there were very few jobs which could be secured for a person who did not read or write. "Big Bill" accepted this as the case and left asking the counselor to keep him in mind if he ever found anything he could do because he wanted to get off welfare.

The counselor talked with a workshop manager in reference to the possibility of employing "Big Bill" as a janitor, if he ever had need of such a person. The fact that he couldn't read or write, and that he was mentally retarded, was explained and the workshop manager said he would like to talk to him and see what could be worked out.

After an interview, the workshop manager decided to give him a try-out as a helper. "Big Bill" surprised everybody, and today he is off welfare and is the custodian for the workshop. He is happy there in his work. He likes to help everyone he can. He takes special pride in keeping the workshop clean and nice looking. "Big Bill" can't read or write, but he is making his own way today.

This particular case is not marked as a successful rehabilitation case, as the case had been closed as "having little potential." This is an example of the fact that sometimes the professionals may be wrong.

SUMMARY

Many more case histories could be written to point out the work of a counselor in this area. It is recognized that much progress has been made in the rehabilitation services for the mentally retarded since the Vocational Rehabilitation Amendments of 1943 made the disability of mental retardation an acceptable one for the program. Workshops, rehabilitation evaluation centers, progress in special education classes and the development of the concept of work-study have all contributed a share to the progress being made. President John F. Kennedy's interest in the field of mental retardation stimulated much research in reference to possible jobs for them. Many gains have been made; however, it is pointed out that most of them have been for the mildly retarded. There is much that needs to be done for those farther down on the scale. There is much need throughout our country for the development of opportunities for those who may not be capable of working in competitive industry. Sheltered workshops must be developed to provide employment on a continuing basis for those who can earn only part of their keep. The development of the type of program needed is a challenge to those working in the field now and to those who will enter this field in the future.

DISCUSSION QUESTIONS

1. Discuss diagnostic information needed for this disability group.
2. Discuss levels of mental retardation and the vocational implications of each level.
3. Discuss special rehabilitation counseling concerns with the mentally retarded.

SUGGESTED READING

Baller, W.R. A study of the present social status of a group of adults who, when they were in elementary schools, were classified as mentally deficient. Genet Psycholog Monogr, 18:165-244, 1936.

Charles, D.C. Ability and accomplishment of persons earlier adjudged mentally deficient. Genet Psycholog Monogr, 4:3-71, 1953.

Clark, G.R., Kivitz, M.S., and Rosen, M. A transitional program for institutionalized adult retarded. Elwyn, Penn. Elwyn Institute, 1968.

Cofer, J.S. An Analysis of vocational failures of mental retardates placed in the community after a period of institutionalization. Am J Ment Def, 65:371-375, 1960.

DiMichael, S.G. (Ed.) New Vocational Pathways for the Mentally Retarded. Washington, D.C., American Personnel and Guidance Association, 5-19, 1966.

Dinger, J.C. Post-school adjustment of former educable retarded pupils. Except Child, 27:353-356, 1961.

Garrett, J.F. Economic benefits of programs for the retarded. Programs for the handicapped, U.S. Department of Health, Education, and Welfare, Secretary's Committee on Mental Retardation, January, 1971.

Gozali, Joav Perception of the EMR special class by former students. Ment Retard, 10:34-35, 1972.

Hardy, Richard E. and Cull, J.G. Readings in Mental Retardation and Physical Disability, Springfield, Thomas, 1974.

Jackson, R.N. Employment adjustment of educable mentally handicapped ex-pupils in Scotland. Am J Ment Def, 72:924-930, 1968.

Joint Report of the President's Committee on Mental Retardation and President's Committee on Employment of the Handicapped. These, too, must be equal: American's needs in habilitation and employment of the mentally retarded. Washington, D.C., 1969.

Miller, E.L. Ability and social adjustment at mid-life of persons earlier judged mentally deficient. Genet Psycholog Monogr, 72:139-198, 1965.

Nixon, R.A. Impact of automation and technological change on employability of the mentally retarded. Am J Ment Def, 75:152-155, 1970.

Phelps, W.R. Attitudes related to the employment of the mentally retarded.

Am J Ment Def, 69:575-585, 1965.

Preparation of mentally retarded youth for gainful employment. U.S. Department of Health, Education, and Welfare, Office of Education, Bulletin 1959, No. 28, Rehabilitation Service Series, No. 507, 20-39.

Stevens, H. and Heber, R., (Eds.) Mental retardation: A review of research. Chicago, University of Chicago Press, 214-259, 1964.

Syden, M. Preparation for work: An aspect of the secondary school's curriculum for mentally retarded youth. Excep Child, 28:325-332, 1962.

Tobias, J. and Gorelick, J. Work characteristics of retarded adults at trainable levels. Ment Retard, 1:338-344, 1963.

Chapter 7

THE VISUALLY IMPAIRED

Psychological Testing Summary
Opinions and Evaluation of Case
Discussion Questions
Suggested Reading

ON May 27, 1964, Ulysses Keystone, age 14, white, male, was referred to Service to the Visually Impaired by a teacher at the School for the Blind for the purpose of receiving Talking Book Service. Ulysses entered the School for the Blind at age 5 and has attended this institution on a continuous basis, presently being in the eighth grade. He was born May 15, 1950 and has resided at his home in Chamberlain during those summer months when he was not in attendance at the School for the Blind.

At the time of referral, the rehabilitation counselor working with this case made the following observation: individual appears to be very self-centered in his thinking processes and unrealistic in terms of his life concepts; for example, individual believes that he is the only blind child in Chamberlain or for that matter in the entire county. It also appears that this individual has led a rather sheltered life during most of his existence.

Family background indicates that Ulysses has three sisters and one brother, all presently living elsewhere with their own established families. The father is a transit construction worker while the mother maintains the household. None of the brothers or sisters have completed college or any other type of specific training, although three of them have spent time in college.

During the next three year period, the agency counselor made occasional contacts with Ulysses during his freshman, sophomore and junior year at the School for the Blind. During this time, the counselor basically offered counseling types of services and did future vocational planning with the client on a somewhat limited basis.

During the latter part of his junior year, Ulysses was given various types of psychological interest and aptitude testing by an educational psychologist at the school. Results with the Wechsler Adult Intelligence Scale (WAIS) yielded a verbal IQ of 114. The results of the verbal portion of the WAIS indicate that the client scored well into the bright range of intelligence. He also was administered the Haptic Intelligence Test for Adult Blind which yielded no average scores. The subject scored low in all areas except arithmetic with an abacus. He was quite successful with this. This appeared to be related to his academic or verbal portion of the Wechsler so that there is this sort of correlation.

Motor Skills Tests administered included the Minnesota Rate of Manipulation and the Pennsylvania Bi-manual Work Sample. The client did not score well in these tests, but did show manipulation skills and did perform them with dexterity even though he was slow and precise. He had good movement and could move from left to right with tasks quite readily; much more so than right to left move.

The examiner felt that practice and training could improve the motor skill area. Results of the California Mental Health Analysis indicated that Ulysses scored low in the following areas: close personal relationships, inter-personal skills, behavior immaturity, emotional instability and feelings of inadequacy. On the other hand, he rated very high in the outlook and goals part of the test.

PSYCHOLOGICAL TESTING SUMMARY

Assets

Mental	Good verbal ability — no real weak areas
	Average or better in all sub-tests
Personal	Really has a high level of aspiration and would like to succeed.
Vocational	Jobs that relate to other people primarily.

Liabilities

Mental	Low in performance areas — slow, really
Physical	Congenitally blind

Personal   Real feelings of inadequacy. This is pointed out in all testing done. He would like to be a professional person. He seems to be afraid to be.

Vocational He is slow in motor skills, though fundamentals are good. Do not recommend outside work, mechanical area, or the sciences. He indicates a definite disinterest in them.

Integration and Interpretation of Test Results

It looks as if this boy could go to college if he wanted to; Vocational school might be appropriate if he is interested. He does have skills that can be trained.

Good intellect generally; good potential in some areas. He wants to succeed, but he is stymied by his own feelings of insecurity and "can I really do it."

Reports indicate that he has few friends. This may be because he hesitates to take the initiative, a kind of fear of self and failure.

Recommendation

This boy needs a good amount of counseling and understanding. There is potential here that should not be allowed to dwindle away. I wouldn't know exactly what steps to take at this time, but I certainly would encourage all the academics he can handle and see if he can't be prepared for a college career. The boy himself suggests General Beadle or Black Hills. Both are probably excellent suggestions.

Try him out for size in counseling sessions; see if he needs some psychological bolstering.

At this time upon first contact, the agency counselor, after doing his initial interview, authorized an eye examination and general physical examination and completed other necessary documentation needed to determine whether this person was eligible for agency service. When the eye report information was received later, it indicated that Ulysses had light perception only in each eye as a result of retro-lental fibroplasia which was caused by an excess of oxygen during time spent in an incubator. Since there was no treatment presently known which could alter a congenital eye condition of this sort, further planning was based on the assumption that vision would never be any better than it was at the present time. During the initial contact with this client, two facts evolved which would be determining factors in any future vocational planning. First, there was an indication that the client needed to remove himself from the home situation and become involved in working on some type of job in order to establish some basic work behavior patterns since he lacked any definable work history. Second, the area of personal adjustment to blindness needed to be worked on intensively, especially in mobility and communications.

During the summer of 1968, Ulysses enrolled at the Evaluation and Training Center in Sioux Falls for the purpose of work adjustment training and personal adjustment to blindness services.

Housing arrangements were procured with the client at the YMCA and the starting date for enrollment was June 2. It had also been determined in planning with the parents that room and board maintenance would have to be provided. The parents were able to contribute to their son's room and board and the agency assisted also.

Results of evaluation and testing after the first five weeks at the Rehabilitation Center resulted in the following observations. The evaluator's assessment was that even though the client's verbal IQ was in the high range, it was difficult for him to conceive that Ulysses could succeed in college. In fact, it was difficult for the evaluator to reach a conclusion regarding any type of successful activity that this client could accomplish. Evaluator's concept of the client was that of being a young child with an adult mind in some areas, but very adolescent in more areas.

The following is an example of one of the evaluations done by Center's staff:

Major Assets

    1. One seems motivated towards employment
    2. Excellent attendance

Problem Areas (Liability)

    1. Unable to accept constructive criticism
    2. At times feels superior to other clients
    3. Somewhat unrealistic as to his own abilities

Progress Since Last Report

1. Has shown little improvement in the reduction in unusual mannerisms
2. Has difficulty retaining a new learned skill without continuous practice

Overall Plan To Be

Identification of a suitable vocational goal

One of the chief concerns was in the area of social acceptability and appropriateness which the evaluator felt was related to the congenital blindness of the client. In fact, the client exhibits many inappropriate social behaviorisms and blindisms.

The Rehabilitation Center's evaluation team also recommended a complete neurological work up which did not indicate any serious neurological difficulties since there was some suspect of brain damage.

One of the key recommendations that was made by the Center's staff was that the client, because of his having led a very sheltered life, be exposed to social experience and different occupational activities which could be obtained outside the home. Also at the time of the initial evaluation it was concluded that about the only potential the client had at that time was vocational placement in a sheltered workshop. It was also recommended that the client receive intensive counseling services along with intensive basic skill training which could possibly produce a higher potential vocational level.

One of the other recommendations that came from the Center's evaluation was that Mr. Keystone is a young man who exhibits considerable ability in verbal intelligence. On the other hand, he exhibits retardation in social skills, work behavior, as well as vocational information and awareness. It appears that the client needs a great deal of encouragement and structuring in terms of nonacademic experiences. It may be advisable to have Mr. Keystone return to the School for the Blind on a post-graduate basis. It is difficult to select area of potential at the present time. There are some indications that Mr. Keystone has some work potential.

Unless he can catch up in his social environment, it is rather difficult to recommend a college plan for him. Areas such as dictaphone, typing, repetitive assembly work, switchboard operation, massage and vending activities should be investigated before a definite vocational plan is developed. Mr. Keystone needs the opportunity to see a counselor on a regular basis in order to talk out problems as well as to have the opportunity to work out structured activities to meet his needs.

Complicating this Center's summary in evaluation was the goal expectation level of the parents, especially the father. The father's insistance that his son must attend and graduate from college was complicated by the fact that three older children in the family had started college and none of them had finished and "at least one of my kids is going to graduate."

In discussing recommendations with the father, his feeling was that independent mobility, correction of inappropriate mannerisms, etc. were not important for success. The father's goal was that his son should first get a college degree and the agency should then place him in a job. He also refused to accept the concept that his son's independence must be a part of his rehabilitation program and job placement.

Although the father indicated that he was absolutely opposed to his son remaining at the Rehabilitation Center for further experience, he did indicate that he would not prevent his son from attending if he so wished.

Ulysses then did return to the Center and spent part of 1968 and most of 1969 at the Center. During this time, he also applied for and received Aid to the Blind. The client at this time, during 1969. expressed an interest in becoming a transcription typist. The plan at that time then was that he would attend the National College of Business in Rapid City starting in the fall of 1969, Also, there was some discussion of a transcription typist program available at Chicago Lighthouse for the Blind. Also the Lighthouse had a program in medical terminology. They also emphasized that at the Chicago Lighthouse, Ulysses would receive much supportive counseling in order to work on minimizing several of the blind mannerisms displayed by him; with the realization that any further placement would be much easier if those mannerisms were reduced to an absolute minimum. When these possibilities were explained to the parents, their interest still centered around the idea of their son attending college although it was rather vague as to what course of study client would pursue if he did attend college.

In November of 1969, it was finally resolved that formal application to the Chicago Lighthouse would be made, which was done. On February 26, 1970, Mr. Keystone officially started a medical transcription program at the Chicago Lighthouse. Ulysses spent a total of 32 weeks at the Chicago Lighthouse and their evaluation reports indicated assets in the area of attendance, motivation and being friendly and personable. They inidcated that the client indicated being anxious in terms of strong organization and retentive ability. Their recommendation after the initial evaluation included: (1) continual induction to dictaphone and typing, (2) enjoys own work and study procedures, (3) weekly group therapy and group discussion, (4) individual counseling as indicated with advisors and instructors.

The client continued to show progress in those areas that needed improvement and he finally completed the course with the following evaluation: grammar and spelling — adequate, typing — 50 WPM, dictaphone — completed dictaphone course and passed the final test with a 142 LPH (minimum score is 125 LPH).

Upon completion of his course even though there were jobs available for the client in the Chicago area, he refused them as he wished to return to his native South Dakota.

His South Dakota counselor became involved in job placement and he returned to Sioux Falls establishing living quarters at the YMCA.

Even though Ulysses had completed his transcription course in December of 1970, the recommendation of the Chicago Lighthouse staff was that he return for further training. Their feeling was that the client could benefit from additional terminology study and should keep up his typing with practice and supervision.

The client, after leaving Chicago on December 1, 1970, spent the remainder of the month visiting relatives at his home in Chamberlain. At the same time an appointment job opening occurred at the Sioux Valley Hospital in Sioux Falls. Mr. Keystone contacted that employer and learned that there was, in fact, no job available even though there was. When the counselor spoke with this employer as to why they had no interview with the client in question, they presented the job in a way which entailed doing many other things other than what the client was trained to do and also expected the individual hired for the job to do some things which would be very difficult for a blind person.

The client then returned to Chicago Lighthouse on January 4 of 1971 to receive additional training. During this time, he did arrange to take the Federal Civil Service test for medical transcription and did pass. The Chicago staff realized that it would be very difficult indeed for the client to find work in South Dakota or any other state while staying in Chicago. It was then agreed that the client would return to Sioux Falls with the idea of making that his base for operation and exploring employment openings in some larger city in South Dakota.

Ulysses spent from January 4 to February 4 (1 month) at the Chicago Lighthouse prior to returning to Sioux Falls. While the client explored employment possibilities, the sheltered workshop within the Rehabilitation Center Facility in Sioux Falls needed an individual with Ulysses' qualifications to do considerable typing of labels, etc. In April of 1971, a possibility of a job opening developed at McKennan Hospital in Sioux Falls but never materialized. A job at the Veterans Administrative Hospital, too, never materialized for him.

It was ascertained at this point that the client needed some assistance in job seeking skills especially in the area of interviewing which he did receive through the Sioux Falls Rehabilitation Center staff. The Center counselor continued to work with the field counselor in the placement process.

During the latter part of May, 1971, the Rehabilitation Center Counselor attended a meeting in Denver and was informed that Fitzsimmons General Hospital was looking for a medical transcription person.

The counselor met with the Director of Civilian Personnel and briefly described Ulysses and his present circumstances and the possibility of placement with their hospital and the current availability of job openings.

On June 1, 1971, the client did, in fact, fly to Denver and interviewed for the position. At this same time, in a cooperative agreement with the Colorado Service to the Visually Impaired, it was agreed that their job placement person work out some of the mechanics in preparation for the interview.

The one concern that the employer had during the interview was the physical ability of the client to handle the position. This matter was sufficiently worked out and the employment position was officially offered to Mr. Keystone. The official starting date of the job then turned out to be June 19. In fact, the client could have started work as early as June 5; however, the details of arranging for house and allowing Ulysses to become familiar with transportation routes, etc. in Denver needed additional time to work out. The placement specialist in Colorado then assisted the client in obtaining housing and also arranged for orientation and mobility training prior to employment.

The client is now successfully employed, having been so for a number of years. His weekly salary at the time of placement was $103.00. He was twenty years old at time of job placement.

OPINIONS AND EVALUATION OF THE CASE

Here we have had an example of a case where the involvement of the client in his own destiny or rehabilitation planning was somewhat tinted by the very strong desire of the parents to, in fact, make all decisions for their son. The agency for other staff constantly had to fight the problem of the father setting a level of expected outcome for the client which, in fact, allowed the client very little involvement in his own rehabilitation and decision making.

The objectivity of the total evaluation process and the use of evaluative instruments was felt to be somewhat less than totally adequate. Some of the most accurate evaluation perhaps took place in actual day to day observation of the client's performance. The reliability and validity of evaluative instruments presently used with blind and severely visually-impaired individuals needs to have some uniformity in terms of use with a blind population.

The area of job placement appeared to be one handled in a

rather loose and haphazard way in that the client himself was given very little assistance in properly preparing himself for an actual job interview. The question that has to be asked is what service could be given to the client in the job placement process which would better assist him assist himself. The gathering of information regarding new job openings in some instances appeared to be incomplete and inconclusive. Also, I think, some of the employers who had jobs available needed to be contacted by an agency person in order to get rid of the blindness barriers that existed in the employer's mind regarding what a blind person can or can not do.

DISCUSSION QUESTIONS

1. Discuss the term "blindness". What is the legal definition? What does it mean?
2. Discuss mobility problems related to partial sight and total blindness.
3. Discuss mobility problems related to vocational decisions.
4. Discuss levels of sensory appreciation among both blind and sighted persons (touch, hearing, etc.).
5. Discuss age of onset of blindness as a factor in adjustment.
6. Discuss sudden blindness and gradual loss of sight as factors in adjustment.

SUGGESTED READING

American Mutual Insurance Alliance, Workers Worth Their Hire. Chicago, Illinois.

American Psychiatric Association Diagnostic and Statistical Manual of Mental Disorders. Washington, D.C., American Psychiatric Association, 1965.

Bauman, Mary K. and Yoder, Norman M. Adjustment to Blindness— Reviewed. Springfield, Thomas, 1966.

Bauman, Mary K. and Yoder, Norman M. Placing the Blind and Visually Handicapped in Professional Occupations. Office of Vocational Rehabilitation, Department of Health, Education, and Welfare, Washington, D.C., 1962.

Carroll, Thomas J. Blindness: What It Is, What It Does, and How to Live With It. Boston, Little, 1961.

Department of Veterans' Benefits, Veterans' Administration They Return to Work. Washington, D.C., U.S. Government Printing Office, 1963.

Hardy, Richard E. Counseling physically handicapped college students. New Outlook for the Blind, 59:182-183, 1965.

Hardy, Richard E. Relating psychological data to job analysis information in vocational counseling. New Outlook for the Blind, 63:202-204, 1969.

Hardy, Richard E. Vocational placement. In Cull, John G. and Hardy, Richard E., Vocational Rehabilitation: Profession and Process. Springfield, Thomas, 1972.

Hardy, Richard E. and Cull, John G. Social and Rehabilitation Services for the Blind. Springfield, Thomas, 1973.

International Society for the Welfare of Cripples Selective Placement of the Handicapped. New York, 1955.

Jones, J.W. Problems in defining and classifying blindness. New Outlook for the Blind, 56:115-121, 1962.

Lofquist, L.H. and Dawis, R.V. Adjustment to Work—A Psychological View of Man's Problems in Work-Oriented Society. New York, Appleton-Century-Crofts, 1967.

Morgan, Clayton A. Personality of counseling. Blindness, AAWB Annual, American Association of Workers for the Blind, Inc. Washington, D.C., 1969.

Chapter 8

THE DIABETIC

Discussion Questions
Suggested Reading

DIABETES is a chronic disease in which the body is unable to make normal use of the sugar in the diet. This condition results from the failure of the pancreas, a gland in the body, to produce a sufficient supply of a hormone called insulin. It is this hormone which enables the body to use sugar.

The seriousness of this disorder varies among individuals. Although there is no known cure for diabetes, the disease can be controlled by drugs, diet and exercise under proper medical supervision. When diabetes is controlled its effects are minimized. In mild cases, diabetes may be controlled by careful regulation of diet and exercise. Many diabetics, however, must take insulin in addition to following prescribed patterns of diet and exercise. Most persons with diabetes participate in the activities associated with normal living. They work, attend school, keep house, travel and engage in sports. There are an estimated 1.7 million persons in the United States with a diagnosis of diabetes. There may be an equal number of persons who have this disease without knowing it.

Vocational rehabilitation services can help persons with diabetes prepare for and find jobs. These services are offered by state vocational rehabilitation agencies. Any disabled person whose disability interfers with his earning a living, holding a job, getting more suitable work, going to school or performing such tasks as keeping house may be helped by vocational rehabilitation.

Services of the vocational rehabilitation agency start with medical determination of the extent of the disability and the disabled person's potential for work. Medical services to reduce the handicap and effects of the disability are arranged, if necessary. Help in choosing the right kind of work is offered by a trained rehabilitation counselor. If a disabled person needs special training for the proper job, this will be provided in a vocational school, college, rehabilitation facility or on the job. Assistance in finding a job may be provided and the rehabilitation counselor helps the disabled person adjust to his new job, if he needs this help.

The aforementioned facts had to be considered by the vocational rehabilitation counselor when Miss Shirley Jones was referred to vocational rehabilitation with a diagnosis of diabetes mellitus, severe. Miss Jones, a 25-year-old, single, Negro female, was referred to vocational rehabilitation by the father of a former rehabilitation client. Prior to the referral, Miss Jones had been employed; however, she had lost her job due to illness. She had to be hospitalized; and at this time, it was discovered that she had diabetes. Upon discharge from the hospital, she was faced with a traumatic decision, "Where do I go from here?" Both of her parents were dead; she had no known living relatives other than a step-grandmother with whom she lived.

She had graduated from high school, and school records indicated above average work. Her past work experience included receptionist for a local doctor and a funeral home. She was very ambitious and had a desire to better herself. She realized that she would have to be trained in order to secure better employment and meet the personal needs brought about by her disability.

An appointment was arranged with the local rehabilitation counselor. The appointment was kept; and at this time, the counselor began to initiate necessary steps in order to determine the client's eligibility for rehabilitation services. Medical information was obtained from the attending physician with the diagnosis being diabetes mellitus, severe, controlled through 40 units of NHU 80 insulin daily and by proper diet and exercise. An evaluation of the applicant's school records, aptitudes, interests and capabilities indicated that her previous employment was grossly inadequate in comparison with her potential. After all information had been gathered, it was determined by the counselor that the client's disability did constitute a substantial handicap; therefore, she was found eligible.

The counselor, at this time, through counseling sessions with the client, began to develop plans of rehabilitation for the client. The client had expressed a desire to enroll in college and obtain a degree in education and become an elementary school teacher. High school records were obtained; they indicated that the client was above average student, and it was determined by the counselor that she could do college work based upon this. However, the biggest task faced by the client and counselor was the fact that the client had no resources in order to enroll in college. Vocational rehabilitation would provide her the maximum services; however, this would not take care of the total cost. This matter was discussed between the counselor and the client, and they agreed that he would contact the college of her choice as to the possibility of a student loan. She was advised by the counselor to go ahead and make application in order that if she should be accepted and could secure a loan or possible employment that by doing this, there would be no delay and she would be able to enroll at the proper time. The client was accepted by the college and received forms to apply for a National Student Defense Loan. Contact was made by the counselor with the coordinator of financial aid at the college. He strongly recommended approval of her application, mentioning the facts of her disability and family background. The client's application for a loan was approved.

At this time, the counselor initiated his plan. The counselor planned to provide the client with the maximum amount in tuition and maintenance as well as drugs which were necessary as a means of helping keep her diabetic condition under control. Her student loan was in the amount of $80 per quarter. This was her total source of income. The counselor realized that it would be quite difficult for the client to meet the needs and demands placed upon students. He counseled with her in regard to this, and he felt that with both of them working together that she would be able to manage and to obtain her degree.

During the course of her training, many problems were encountered. Food at the student cafeteria was not appropriate for her restricted diet. Also, she had to take insulin at regular intervals, therefore, she had to keep a supply on hand, which had to be stored in a refrigerator which was not available. Therefore, it was necessary for the client to secure housing off campus.

Before the fall quarter of her junior year, the client came by the counselor's office and informed him that the college had refused to grant her a loan for that year due to the limited amount of funds available. The client had received this loan for her first two years and had maintained above average grades during this time. The counselor felt that because of the client's financial situation the college should be notified about all of the client's circumstances and needs. The counselor contacted the coordinator of financial aid at the college and explained to him the details about the client. The coordinator assured the counselor at this time that he would contact the client and stated that he would get her in school one way or another. The following day, the client called the counselor to let him know that she had gotten a loan from the school for $300 for the next year. The client was able to continue with her education and completed her work for her degree.

Upon graduation from college, she was employed in the Jackson Public School System earning $580 per month. Followup with the client was made and the counselor continued to encourage the client to stay under the care of her doctor for frequent checkups, continue on her medication and eat the proper diet. The counselor contacted all interested parties and informed them of the client's progress and of the fact that she had completed her college work, obtained her degree, was now employed and that her case was being closed in Status 26 rehabilitated.

I feel that this was a very good case and much evidence was displayed by the counselor and the client in planning the objective. Counseling and guidance was a very important service rendered; many obstacles were presented, but through wise decisions and careful planning, these obstacles were overcome and the client is now a productive citizen, contributing to the welfare of society.

DISCUSSION QUESTIONS

1. Discuss the medical implication in terms of vocational selection for the diabetic individual. (What types of industrial employment should be avoided by persons who are diabetic?)

2. Discuss the effects of too much or too little insulin.

SUGGESTED READING

Best, C.H. and Taylor, N.B. Physiological Basis of Medical Practice, 5th Ed., Baltimore, Williams & Wilkins Co., 1950.

Cull, J. G. and Hardy, R. E. Counseling and Rehabilitating the Diabetic, Springfield: Charles C Thomas, 1974.

Felton, J.S., Perkins, D.C. and Lewin, M. A Survey of Medicine and Medical Practice for the Rehabilitation Counselor, Washington, D.C.: V.R.A., Department of Health, Education, and Welfare, 1966.

Hardy, R.E. and Cull, J.G. Severe Disabilities: Social and Rehabilitation Approaches, Springfield, Thomas, 1973.

U.S. Department of Health, Education, and Welfare, Public Health Service, Diabetes Source Book, Publication No. 1168, Washington, D.C. Government Printing Office, 1968.

Wright, B.A. Physical Disability — A Psychological Approach, New York, Harper & Row, 1960.

Wright, B.A. "Some Problems, Some Concepts, and Some Solutions", In A. Sales (Ed.) Supervision of Rehabilitation Counseling Contacts: Selected Psychological Considerations, Emporia, Kansas: Kansas State Teachers College Press, 1971.

Chapter 9

THE BLIND DIABETIC

Description of Case
Summary
Psychological Testing
Summary
Conclusion
Discussion Questions
Suggested Reading

CLEM Marlborro, age 26, white, male, was referred to an agency by his mother on September 21, 1966. His mother was apparently a bit confused between the State Service to the Blind and State School for the Blind, thinking that the School for the Blind was part of the agency service. The initial referral question concerned itself with the mother wanting to locate some type of schooling (educational) service for her son, indicating she said, "my son just can't make up his mind what to do." Mrs. Marlborro asked the agency for information concerning what courses are taught at the School for the Blind, how long in duration and if this would be the place for her son to get some type of care and diet since she indicated her son had severe diabetes.

Also involved in the referral of this young man was the local Lions Club which also directed a letter to the director of the agency indicating that their Lions Club was doing some investigation for a young man in their area who had lost his eye sight through a diabetic condition. They, as did the mother, requested information concerning the School for the Blind and asked whether the agency paid for room, board, tuition and other fees. They also indicated in their referral letter that the client was sensitive about his eye condition and also that he was presently living on a farm with his brother and did enjoy that type of work.

The agency counselor first made contact with the client on February 4, 1967.

DESCRIPTION OF CASE

Mr. Marlborro, age 27, is a high school graduate having graduated from Lemmon High School, Lemmon, South Dakota, in June of 1959. His favorite subjects were science, biology and speech. He disliked algebra. He is single and from June 1, 1959 to March of 1966 has worked on shares with his brother at Meadow, South Dakota, as rancher-farmer. Prior to that time, he had worked at construction work and for other ranchers in the area. After he lost vision in one eye in March of 1966, he lived with his mother who is a widow in Lemmon. He was under the care of an ophthalmologist in Rapid City and a short time after March lost most of the vision in the second eye. At this time, he did go to Boston to a diabetes clinic and also contacted specialists at Rochester where he was told that nothing could be done for his vision. He has been a diabetic for four years and claims that his diabetes is under control. Mr. Marlborro stated that he had never been happy living in town and always lived and worked on a farm. Prior to his blindness, he share-farmed with his brother. His plans as of this contact report were to enter into a dairying operation with his brother since he had already built a dairy barn and purchased a cream separator. He planned on starting to farm in the spring having initially purchased seven or eight head of cows.

Further discussion took place concerning mechanics of the farming operation. It is important to note that at this time in his vocational planning, plans for farming were very important. The agency counselor felt that the client had an acceptable attitude toward his blindness and learned that the client has difficulty traveling in strange surroundings and has had some adjustment problems. The counselor suggested that the client attend an adjustment center recommending Minneapolis Society for the Blind. Both the mother and the client were in favor of this suggestion, but wanted a time delay until he could get started in his dairying project. The client was very eager at this time to start moving in some direction as he had been sitting around for some time.

The counselor suggested in counseling that the client attempt to attend the Rehabilitation Center as soon as possible since delaying this training would only hold back the client's total adjustment to blindness. In other words, the client wants to attend the Rehabilitation Center, desires independence, wants to learn Braille, but also wants to start on his dairy project. He did indicate that he preferred the Rehabilitation Center in Minneapolis, since he had a sister living there.

The counselor completed necessary completion of survey forms and authorized appropriate general medical and eye examination along with explaining the services of the agency.

The counselor later contacted the local welfare office and stated that the case worker there was very concerned about Mr. Marlborro. The case worker stated that after Mr. Marlborro went blind, he shut himself off from all others and was still isolating himself from his friends. The welfare office was approached both by the mother and the local Lions Club who had some concern about the client's isolation and general attitude.

Further discussion indicated that the local Lions Club was willing to pay a share of Clem's expenses while he attended the rehabilitation center.

The next contact was on August 27, 1967. Contact indicated Mr. Marlborro was still interested in attending the Rehabilitation Center and at the same time the counselor described another Rehabilitation Center which is located in Little Rock, Arkansas. The client discussed in some detail some of the problems he was having with his sight in that during the day his travel vision was functional, but once it became dark, he would get lost.

Further detailed discussion took place concerning techniques the client used in his farming operation in general.

Mr. Marlborro then discussed in detail how he would get to a Rehabilitation Center, and the counselor explained the procedure. The counselor's impression at this point is that even though the client knows he needs the services offered at a Rehabilitation Center, that as long as things are going fairly well at home, there will continue to be some delay.

The next contact with the client was on October 20, 1967 by letter. In the letter the counselor simply asked Mr. Marlborro which rehabilitation facility he had decided he would attend and indicated the cost of attending both. The counselor then asked the client to respond.

By telephone contact it was resolved that Mr. Marlborro would be attending the Minneapolis Society for the Blind with an approximate starting date of November 5, 1967. Letter of referral and appropriate referral information was sent to the Minneapolis Society for the Blind staff. Information sent included a brief case history and requested type of training. Specifically, intensive training in the area of mobility and orientation, Braille and other adjustment to blindness services were requested. Also some concern about the client's general diabetic condition and control was indicated. The client was again contacted on a personal visit on November 4, 1967. During this contact, the mechanics of assisting him in his journey to Minneapolis were discussed and worked out. The client also discussed in considerable detail why he had chosen Minneapolis in lieu of Little Rock. His reasoning was that Little Rock was too far away and that his decision to attend the Minneapolis Rehabilitation Center was greatly influenced by his sister's impression of that facility. He at this time indicated an interest in investigating the field of piano tuning.

He officially entered the Minneapolis Society for the Blind on November 9, 1967 and spent until March, 1968 at this facility (four months).

During his progress at Mineapolis Society for the Blind, the following types of services were offered; teaching of Braille, typing, home economics, orientation of mobility, physical condition, activities of daily living and psychological testing and considerable counseling.

During this period of time, Mr. Marlborro met and became engaged to a 21-year-old girl who is fully sighted. He had known her since December and had been dating her for about six weeks. He felt that his fiancee had "a better understanding of him and his condition than others he had previously dated." By this he meant that when the occasion presented itself, he talked with her about his visual impairment and diabetes and the limitations this condition would of necessity impose on both of them. Only after he felt that she fully understood and accepted them, did he propose marriage. Their plans at this time involved becoming married in September of 1968.

A summary of his initial evaluation at the Rehabilitation Center in the various areas indicated the following: Typing, completed the basic aspects of the course and showed constant and steady improvement; Home Economics, greatly motivated towards self-care with good comprehension of instruction and manual coordination; Orientation Mobility, remaining vision of assistance to him in inside building and in foot travel; anxious to learn cane technique but has some difficulty in accepting it because of his remaining vision, but voiced objection to the use of a cane in his own home town: the blindfold was used, and the client cooperated well, motivated with good comprehension ability and above average progress; Physical Conditioning, took an active part and was well-motivated; Occupational Therapy, quickly completed the entire activities of living.

SUMMARY

In general, the Rehabilitation Center was very pleased with the client's progress and stated he was a morale builder in the groups because of his quiet way. He is quite a popular and significant member of the student group. The center's staff felt that he would become more accepting of the use of a white cane for travel as time went by.

PSYCHOLOGICAL TESTING

General Observations: Quite apprehensive about the tests he was to take expressing particular concern about the "IQ Test," since he felt the results would determine whether he would go to college or not. Spoke quite easily and readily about his background and said that he was currently considering a change from the ranching he had been engaged in. He has written to three or four colleges and asked for material on entrance requirements, etc. Said he wanted to "work with people," but did not seem definite about the particular field this might involve. Attitude generally responsive, pleasant and cooperative, although anxious throughout the examination.

Wechsler Adult Intelligence Test

The verbal portion of the Wechsler Adult Intelligence skill yielded a verbal IQ of 109. The performance half of the test was not administered due to client's visual handicap. The strong vocational test for men administered indicated the following:

> Interest appeared most similar to those of veterinarians, farmers, vocational, agricultural teachers, forest service — public administrator, social science, high school teacher, and musician. Interest appeared consistent with general background. Does not have any clear pattern of interest, although he does express a dislike for the physical sciences. Interest to resemble, to a lesser degree, those persons engaged in social service types of occupation.

Minnesota Multiphasic Personality Inventory

He experienced no difficulty with the mechanics of the test, but did tend to be quite defensive in answering the items. Although the resulting profile must be interpreted with caution, he does indicate anxiety, feelings of inadequacy and excessive worry. He feels doubtful in his own ability to live up to the expectations other people have for him and hence feels apprehensive and insecure and can be expected to have difficulty in establishing close personal relationships with the people. A counselor in working with him might find him rather resistant to changing or developing clinically useful dependence. When stress situations become too threatening, he might be expected to develop some outing with behavior. The prcfile would raise some question about the maximal scholastic or vocational level this man would be motivated to attain.

Results of Audiogram

Results of testing indicated a hearing loss in the right ear; a 4000 – 8000 decibel range.

SUMMARY

Mr. Marlborro is a 28-yearold man who has been operating a

small ranching project, but is currently interested in attending college. Although he obtained a verbal IQ of 109, this is probably not a good estimate of his intelligence which could be better described as being quite normal. He was quite anxious throughout the entire test situation and this anxiety did appear to transfer with his performance. Despite his statement that he is most interested in "working with people," his high scores on the interest test were in the occupations of farming and vocational-agriculture teacher. His current interest in "working with people" might be a partial review of his former employment or a reflection of the environment he experienced while in Minneapolis. If he does desire further education, the possibility of advanced training in agricultural types of activities might be considered. Since "success" seems so important to this man, his chances of success will probably be greater in a nonacademic curriculum.

Since reports from the Minneapolis Society for the Blind indicate that Mr. Marlborro's manual dexterity is above average and since information of this kind would not seem particularly useful, this aspect was not further investigated.

After the client's experience at the Rehabilitation facility in Minneapolis, he returned to his place of business at Meadow, South Dakota.

Contact Report of April 7, 1968

The report indicated that the field counselor did considerable counseling with the client in terms of his decision to attend Black Hills State College in the fall. He has decided to major in social work. Considerable discussion also took place concerning the possibility of pre-marital counseling for both the client and his fiancee since the wedding was now definitely planned for September.

Contact Report of June 16, 1968

The agency counselor again discussed with the client upcoming college plans and, in fact, with the client visited the educational facility. The counselor assisted the client in the location of suitable housing and also counseled with client concerning the possibility of his exploring part-time employment along with the possibility that his wife might seek employment.

Contact Report of August 10, 1968

The counselor learned about contacting the client that he and his fiancee had, in fact, gotten married on July 22. The client and his wife were planning on moving to Spearfish by August 16, in order to start school.

Contact Report of September 8, 1968

The counselor contacted the client and his wife at their apartment which they are very happy with and occupied on September 5. College registration was September 6, and the client attended his first class on September 7. The counselor worked with him in learning to operate a tape recorder which the counselor left with the client. At the same time, the client indicated that he had received his first Aid to the Blind check on September 7, of which has been part of prior planning in order to meet college expenses. Also, the counselor discussed "Readers Service" with the client, which is available from the agency and other expenses including insurance, etc.

Contact Report of October 27, 1968

General things were discussed in terms of progress taking place in school. He indicated that mid term grades were as follows:
biology – A; English – B; sociology – C; under graduate course – B

Contact Report of January 18, 1969

The counselor and client discussed grades received there in the fall quarter's performance. He was quite disturbed over the fact that he got a "C" in sociology, his major. He is to take the following subjects beginning second semester: physical science,

English, family relations and economics for a total of 14 quarter hours. The registrar had recommended to the client that he take 17 hours during the semester, but had trouble scheduling an additional three hours.

Contact Report of March 14, 1969

The counselor found that Mr. Marlborro had received two (C's), two (B's), and one (A), for past quarter's work. He plans on taking 17 hours this coming quarter in subject areas related to his major.

Contact Report of May 8th and 17th, 1969

The client and his wife are expecting a baby, and the counselor continues to work with budget consideration.

Contact Report of March 14 thru August 1, 1969

The Marlborros are awaiting the arrival of their first child. Mr. Marlborro is having considerable health problems with his diabetic condition and his remaining sight is rapidly failing. His wife states that he had refused to see a doctor or get an eye examination. The counselor authorized a blood sugar test and an eye examination. In May, Mr. Marlborro saw an opthalmologist, Doctor Palmerton, who assisted the client to better understand his eye condition. Results of the test indicated that the blood sugar level was somewhat high. The Client started on a new Acidity Urine Test and intensive Sugar Urine Test. The client appears to have a better understanding of his diabetes condition and is seeing the doctor on a regular basis. In August, the counselor received a call from Mr. Marlborro concerning severe pain in his left eye (the one with the diabetic cataract). The client saw the doctor and the pain was relieved by medication.

Contact Report of September 5, 1969 thru March 22, 1970

The client was having less difficulty with pain in his eye as medication is keeping tension down. He also indicated that if pain develops again that he would consider having the eye removed.

On March 22, Mr. Marlborro stated that he was having a bit of trouble with pain in his eye and that he would probably have surgery as soon as school was out.

Eye Diagnosis

Light perception only — both eyes percentage loss with best correction 100 percent (100%) both eyes.

Diagnosis Bilateral — extensive retinitis proliferans and retinal detachments. Primary and contributory cause of eye pathology is diabetes mellitus.

On April 23, 1969, Mr. Marlborro was examined by Dr. K. M. Illig, Pierre Ophthalmologist because of a glaucoma condition. Doctor Illig recommended a tube implant procedure and arrangements were made for this operation. Dr. Illig provided the surgery at no cost and the agency rendered financial assistance with the hospitalization and office calls for post-operative care. Mr. Marlborro entered the hospital on May 25 and surgery was performed on May 29, 1969. The tube implant was successful to the extent that it worked satisfactorily. However, due to a problem of having too many skin flaps over the tube, it only did 50 percent of the work. It was, therefore, necessary to have a second tube implant which was done in late June. Mr. Marlborro was released from the hospital on July 6, 1969. During this time it also became known that Mrs. Marlborro was pregnant which made the Department of Public Welfare field worker somewhat unhappy. The counselor also discussed with the Department of Public Welfare field worker the fact that Mr. Marlborro had expressed interest in obtaining his M.A. Degree. The department of Public Welfare worker informed counselor that once Clem finished his four years of college his Aid to Dependent Children would be cut. The counselor made no attempt at this time to press the point with the Department of Public Welfare worker. Mr. Marlborro's grades at this time appeared very satisfactory with the exception of earning a slightly lower grade than he had wanted in sociology which was his major.

Contact Report of August 20 thru September 19, 1969

It was learned that the second tube implant procedure was unsuccessful. Dr. Illig reported that there was a skin growth behind the pupil which prevented fluid from getting to the tubes. He proposed to cut a hole in the iris — making it possible for the fluid to reach the tubes and thus allow drainage to take place. If this operation was not successful, the eye would have to be enucleated. This was explained to Mr. Marlborro who agreed to attempt the procedure regardless. He received surgery on August 26, which was apparently successful and Mr. Marlborro returned to college in time to register for the fall quarter.

Contact Report of October – November, 1969

Mr. Marlborro reported to the counselor that grades were coming along well and that his eyes seemed to be alright after the last operation. At this time the case was transferred from the original rehabilitation counselor to a newly assigned counselor without incident. Mrs. Marlborro gave birth to their second child during this period, also making the Welfare Director serving that area somewhat unhappy.

Contact Report of February 28, 1969

Clem reports no particular concerns with his schooling or scholastic work in general. At this time and on previous occasions, Mr. Marlborro had expressed some interest in attending graduate school for study. In later discussions with Mrs. Marlborro, it was reported that her husband, Clem, was afraid of graduate school and that the only reason he had gone as far as he had in his college training was because he felt this is what the counselor of this agency wanted. She stated that Mr. Marlborro would have been happier had he remained in a farm project. Considerable discussion followed this contact and the client was to consider and explore further possibilities in the area of attending graduate school.

Contact Report of May-June, 1970

Mr. Marlborro's scholastic work progressing satisfactorily during this time. It became evident, however, that his problem with glaucoma was again serious. The second tube implant by Dr. Illig apparently was not successful and it became necessary for Mr. Marlborro to take medication to control his pressure throughout the summer semester. The family was now and had been for a period of time, recipients of Aid to Dependent Children payments and the process of persuading the Department of Public Welfare officials to continue this aid should Mr. Marlborro decide to attend graduate school was begun.

Contact Report of August-September, 1970

Mr. Marlborro registered for fall term at BHTC as authorized by the agency. He managed to take enough electives in history so that he would have a history as well as a social science major.

Contact Reports of October 4 thru December 18, 1970

Mr. Marlborro, through long discussions with his immediate family came to the decision that it would be perhaps best to hold off to attend graduate school at this time in his life. His goal at this point was that upon completion of his degree that he would seek employment either with the school system or state and or federal government.

During this contact, the agency counselor also received information to the effect that Mr. Marlborro was not keeping himself in complete control from a diabetic standpoint. This situation was discussed especially with the wife, who indicated that her husband did take an occasional supplemental shot of insulin when he feels he should. The counselor suggested to the Marlborros that a doctor should be seen as soon as possible so that the diabetic condition could be put in proper control.

Contact Report of March 24, 1971

Considerable discussion took place between counselor and client concerning his doing practice teaching in the Lab School during the upcoming summer months which will allow him to receive his teaching certificate; therefore, allowing him to start teaching in the fall of 1971.

The client reported that school was proceeding on schedule with no serious problems. The client discusses and shows some concern about having the family's ADC cut off once he begins employment.

Contact Report of June 23, 1971

The counselor contacted Mr. Marlborro at home and found that he is getting along satisfactorily with his practice teaching and has not experienced any great difficulty. Mr. Marlborro states that he is using his Braille more now than in the past since he will be administering his first test in a couple of days. The client reports that he has been in contact with personnel officials at the Veterans' Hospital in Fort Meade concerning the possibility of obtaining a position as a social worker's aide. Fort Meade advised Mr. Marlborro to contact the Veterans' Hospital in Cheyenne, Wyoming, as that hospital is reportedly considering adding such a person to their staff.

Contact Report of August 6, 1971

Mr. Marlborro called the state director advising him that his family had to move to another location which would cost more money. Because of this added cost, the welfare department is giving consideration to increasing his rent proportionately and was reinstating his wife's ADC payments to include the amount of Readers Service paid by the agency. Mr. Marlborro was advised that the agency could not provide maintenance unless the client was receiving or engaged in a training program or for the first month of his placement. He was advised that the agency did pay their trips necessary during the placement process. Mr. Marlborro stated to director that he actually enjoyed teaching as he said, "It kind of gets in your blood." Mr. Marlborro has made an additional application for a special education position in the Cheyenne area and the prospect looks good. The director suggested that he contact the director of the Wyoming program for additional recommendation. Mr. Marlborro also has an application in for a rehabilitation counselor position with the Oregon Commission for the Blind. The client has also made application with the state of Oklahoma.

Contact Report of October 26, 1971

Mr. Marlborro reports that he has now completed his college training including the practice teaching without undue difficulty. He also states that he has been in contact with the St. Paul Rehabilitation Center regarding a job in rehabilitation of the unemployed, displaced by mechanization and job change. He and his family are presently living on ADC benefits which allows him only enough money for basic necessities. The client had made contact with many agencies including the State Employment Service, the Department of Public Welfare and similar agencies within the state and outside the state. As yet he has found nothing. The client was assured that the agency would do everything that was possible in the way of assisting him in his attempt to secure employment.

Contact Report of January 22, 1972

The State Employment Office in Rapid City reports that Mr. Marlborro has taken a Civil Service Test of some kind in Minnesota and that he passed. They were unable to provide information as to what the test was for and what, if any, employment possibilities have resulted from it. Mr. Marlborro should be contacted by counselors of agency in the Black Hills area in order to assist and keep abreast of job development.

Contact Report of March 30 – April 27, 1972

On this date the counselor was advised by Mr. Marlborro that he was attempting to obtain employment as a teacher in the Bison Public School System. The client states that one of the board members is a friend of the Marlborro family and that this board member was assisting the client in the placement process. The counselor suggested to the client that he place his name with the Personnel Referral Service of the American Foundation for the Blind. The client was advised that he should contact the superintendent of the Redfield State School and Hospital concerning possible openings. The client was very much concerned that he had not yet found employment. Mr. Marlborro stated that, "I don't enjoy sitting around and doing nothing, as it is not good for my health." On April 14, the client received a telephone call from the agency director indicating that the North Dakota School for the Blind had need for a teacher of Braille.

Mr. Marlborro stated at this time that he had been informed that he would receive a contract with the Bison Public School System and that if the term was satisfactory, he would accept a position there. He stated that he would only have to teach history, government and social studies. Mr. Marlborro reported that his starting salary would be $4600 per year, but he was uncertain as to other terms of the contract. On April 27, Mr. Marlborro telephoned the counselor indicating that he had received and, in fact, signed the contract at a salary of $4659 per year. The salary is to be paid in twelve monthly payments of $387.50 less all withholding taxes. No summer month employment will be expected by the school. Teaching will be done on the secondary level which consisted of approximately sixty to eighty students. The contract was signed and returned to the Bison Public School on May 1, 1972.

Follow-up Contact of November 11, 1972

The counselor contacted the client at his home in Bison, South Dakota and learned that he was satisfactorily employed in a field that he truly enjoyed and was completely satisfied with his work. The client remarked that in addition to his regular teaching duties, he had also been doing some counseling for the superintendent. He enjoys this immensely and hopes to continue doing some work in this area. The client informed the counselor that he feels he has found a permanent place in society and that he will continue in this field. He feels that his job is permanent and that all persons connected with the position were satisfied. The cient is happy with his present salary and feels confident he will be offered a contract next year at which time he expects to ask for an increase of $300 — $500 per year. The client remarked that he may move to a larger school in two to three years. The counselor informed him that agency would be most happy to assist him at such time if he thought it necessary.

Medical and Follow-up Contact of January 17, 1973

On the date previous to this contact, Dr. K. M. Illig, Pierre Ophthalmologist, telephoned the counselor. Doctor Illig stated that previously he had had a discussion with Mr. Marlborro and mentioned that the glaucoma condition had worsened and that his eye was quite painful. The Counselor contacted Mr. Marlborro who then reported that approximately three weeks ago he had been hospitalized by Dr. E. S. Palmerton of Rapid City and had the eye eneucleated with a moveable implant globe installed. The client also stated that there was some post-surgical reaction in that he had been hospitalized, but that he was now quite alright. He stated that he will be getting the prosthesis in the very near future and the eneucleation procedure had made it possible for him to continue with his teaching. Mr. Marlborro inquired as to approximate cost of the operation and counselor advised that this type of operation is listed at about $200. Mr. Marlborro stated that this is not covered by insurance, but that he would be able to work out the payment satisfactorily.

Case officially closed as of February 23, 1973.

CONCLUSION

The critical problem that existed in this case throughout was that of the diabetes and lack of control. The concern of the agency staff throughout was the final dehabilitating effect that the diabetes would have in terms of breaking down the major body systems and, in fact, possibly causing death. Also evident was that for a time the client exhibited lack of concern and self-discipline in the control of his own diabetic regime. Only after some very traumatic turn of events in terms of the client's eye condition did he then realize the seriousness of his general diabetic condition. The question that could be asked would be what type of counsel did the people reporting the various medical disciplines give this client in terms of the potential seriousness of his condition. Again in the area of vocational planning, the objectivity of the evaluative instruments that were used could be questioned considering the final vocational outcome; for example, the field of social work as a vocational goal was contraindicated by the psychological testing results.

In this case extreme directness by the counselor in his counseling procedure while working with this individual in his total rehabilitation allowed the client minimal involvement and input into his own rehabilitation.

DISCUSSION QUESTIONS

1. What vocational areas should be avoided by the blind diabetic?
2. What are the medical implications for vocational choice among blind diabetic persons?
3. What special problems does paraphernalia bring to the diabetic who is blind?

SUGGESTED READING

Best, C.H. and Taylor, N.B. Physiological Basis of Medical Practice, 5th Ed., Baltimore, Williams & Wilkins Company, 1950.

Cull, J.G. and Hardy, R.E. Counseling and Rehabilitating the Diabetic. Springfield: Charles C Thomas, 1974.

Felton, J.S., Perkins, D.C, and Lewin, M. A Survey of Medicine and Medical Practice for the Rehabilitation Counselor, Washington, D.C., V.R.A., Department of Health, Education and Welfare, 1966.

Hardy, R.E. and Cull, J.G. Social and Rehabilitation Services for the Blind. Springfield, Thomas, 1972.

Hardy, R.E. and Cull, J.G. Severe Disabilities: Social and Rehabilitation Approaches. Springfield, Thomas, 1973.

U.S. Department of Health, Education, and Welfare, Public Health Service, Diabetes Source Book, Publication No. 1168, Washington, D.C., U.S. Government Printing Office, 1968.

Wright, B.A. Physical Disability — A Psychological Approach, New York, Harper & Row, 1960.

Wright, B.A. "Some Problems, Some Concepts, and Some Solutions" In A Sales (Ed.) Supervision of Rehabilitation Counseling Contacts: Selected Psychological Considerations, Emporia, Kansas, Kansas State Teachers College Press, 1971.

Chapter 10

CANCER

Cancer: Liposarcoma Resulting in Hemipelvectomy
Discussion Questions
Suggested Reading

CANCER consists of a group of diseases that afflict men and animals. Cancers, which can develop in any organ or tissue of the body, are abnormal new growths. These growths may invade and destroy surrounding normal tissues, or they may set up secondary colonies in distant parts of the body. Malignant growths are composed of cancerous cells which differ from normal cells in many ways, not all of them yet known.

Neurofibromatosis, von Recklinhausen's disease, is a developmental disease of unknown cause characterized by multiple tumors of the peripheral nerves, cranial nerves and skin and associated with circumscribed patches of pigment. The disease is often familial, inherited as an autosomal dominant trait. The disease is rarely fatal except in those who develop sarcamatous degeneration; the prognosis should be guarded, however, since intraspinal or intracranial tumor can cause death.

Vocational rehabilitation services can help many former cancer patients regain a high degree of self-sufficiency. This may involve the selection of new occupations, training or other preparations required by new lines of work.

The aforementioned medical data were considered by the vocational rehabilitation counselor when John Smith was referred to vocational rehabilitation for vocational rehabilitation services. The subject had previously received training through vocational rehabilitation as a bookkeeper based upon his disability of neurofibromatosis with severe scoliosis. John currently has multiple disabilities (1) von Recklinhausen's Disease (2) Sarcomatous degeneration of a neurofibromatosis (3) congenital heart disease, ASD, paroxysmal atrial tachycardia, Grade I.

Further diagnostic work uncovered the fact that the subject was anemic. Although the prognosis for the subject's primary disabling condition at this time was guarded with prospects for life expectancy beyond several years doubtful, it was decided to accept the applicant as a client and to provide needed vocational rehabilitation services to hopefully return him to employment as an offset printer for a state governmental agency. The subject's youth, vocational and demonstrated determination, drive and optimism carried much weight in the counselor's arriving at a decision of eligibility. Upon establishment of the applicant's eligibility for additional vocational rehabilitation services, a plan of services was developed and initiated. The rehabilitation plan was to provide physical restoration services (evacuation of a hematoma), medication to alleviate the subject's anemic condition and an appliance in the form of a new cellulose acetate jacket.

Following an extended period of hospitalization, the subject was released to the care of his private physician. Counseling and guidance services were found to be needed and were provided throughout this period of time. Concentrated, extensive counseling sessions were necessary in order to assist the client to identify and accept his multiplicity of impairments. As soon as the subject's physical condition would permit, he was measured for the aforementioned cellulose acetate jacket. Construction of the jacket took some several weeks. Upon its completion and proper fitting, the subject and the rehabilitation counselor met concerning his satisfaction with the jacket and other physical restoration services rendered him by vocational rehabilitation. The client expressed satisfaction with the jacket and other services rendered him by the agency. The subject subsequently returned to his employment as an offset printer with a state governmental agency. He later was promoted to and is currently functioning as the official head of that department with annual earnings of $6792. The subject's cancerous condition (sarcomatous degeneration of a neurofibromatosis) appears to have either stabilized, been arrested or actually be progressing at a much slower rate than originally anticipated from a medical standpoint. The rehabilitation counselor feels that the subject's mental attitude, which is very positive and all pervasive, contributes greatly to the fact that he is functioning adequately both physically and vocationally. Although the case has been officially closed in Status 26 as rehabilitated, the counselor continues to enjoy a good relationship with the client, leaving the door open for continued counseling and supportive therapy if the need for such is indicated.

It is felt that the subject's vocation is in keeping with his capabilities especially in view of his recent promotion. He appears to have made an adequate psychological adjustment to his terminal disease and its myriad of ramifications, from both personal and societal perspectives. He continues to present a pleasant, gregarious, viable personality and to maintain meaningful relationships with friends, relatives and peers.

Mr. Smith's longevity has exceeded medical prognosis by some two years. He exudes optimism, zeal and enthusiasm to such high degrees that they appear to have either arrested, retarded or precluded despritualization and surrender to his usual lethal physical malady. Although an exacerbation of his condition could recur at any time, the involved vocational rehabilitation counselor feels that the subject has the courage and spirit to combat such an eventuality. Although single, Mr. Smith maintains a warm and close relationship with his family.

In exploring positive character traits, one would do well to utilize Mr. Smith as a subject. His demonstrated determination, courage and lust for life would certainly qualify him for such a choice.

CANCER: LIPOSARCOMA
RESULTING IN HEMIPELVECTOMY

One day in mid 1966, Arthur Craig discovered a bump on the back of his thigh just above the knee joint. His doctor advised that it was a "fatty tumor" usually non-malignant, but should be removed if it caused any discomfort, so arrangements were made to remove it November 1966.

The doctor reported that the tumor was about the size of a large orange, and since it "didn't look too good," took more of the area around it than originally planned. Pathology reports identified it as a liposarcoma, and ten daily X-ray treatments were prescribed with good results. It was the opinion of the surgeon through periodic followup examinations that the growth had been completely removed.

By 1970, at age 49, Art and his wife, Claire, both with good jobs as an accountant and secretary and rearing seven children, were happy and confident that this medical problem was behind them and that after 25 years of work and planning they were going to finish the new home they were building in a nice area and give their children an even better environment of ambition and hope. Their oldest son was already in college and a daughter was to start in the fall. The youngest boy was eight.

On April 13, 1970, Art was showering after having worked till late at night to make ready this "dream home," when he noticed a small lump behind his left knee. The shock was electrifying, and you can imagine the anguish as the husband and wife talked of this dark discovery. There was not much rest that night for them.

An appointment was again made with the doctor. A biopsy was scheduled and the entire tumor removed. It was not quite as big as the first one, but also found to be a liposarcoma in the same location.

The tumor clinic recommended a hemipelvectomy amputation.

This shocking reality was difficult to accept and the patient sought confirming consultation at the Mayo Clinic. His doctor made arrangements in early May, and the head of the Mayo Tumor Clinic conducted tests and consultations for three days. The results showed the patient in excellent physical condition generally, but physicians concurred with the recommendation for a hemipelvectomy immediately as the only course of action. The patient thought, "Doctors recommend, but the final word must come from the patient — go ahead and amputate. Cancer can kill and amputation is the gateway to a little different kind of life. But there is really no other sensible choice."

Upon his return home, Art was referred to a general surgeon who explained every aspect of the situation, including the use of a prosthesis (as the Mayo doctors had also done) and the left hemipelvectomy was scheduled for May 15, with Art's own doctor assisting. The operation was a complete success. No further spreading of the cancer was noted, and after several days in intensive care, Art moved to his regular room. At first he felt like his amputated leg was sticking up at a 45° angle and he couldn't do a thing about it. Much later the phantom pain and phantom sensation tended to disappear except on extensive, continuous wearing of his prosthesis.

Physical therapy began four days post-operatively on the tilt table, going the full 90° upright and using pulley weights, sand bags and dumbbells for arm exercise. He progressed to hopping between the parallel bars and learning how to get down from the cart and to the floor and back with little or no help. He could not use a wheel chair because sitting was too painful at this time from scar tenderness and the strain of holding his balance due to loss of tissue causing a roll to one side. This was to be remedied when a prosthesis is worn.

After a week or so, Art was fitted with crutches and given ample opportunity to become accustomed to them before being shown how to go up and down steps. Later he was allowed to take the crutches back to his room from P.T. and could take walks in the hall if someone were available to walk with him holding a safety belt in addition to walking with crutches during the P.T. sessions twice a day. It became boring, and the waiting on the cart before and after P.T. sessions to return to his room was worse.

During this time, the limb company representative visited Art and left some pamphlets, including a picture of the type of prosthesis that he would eventually use. This salesman, an above-knee amputee himself, was very helpful and understanding in talking with Art and made a formal referral to the Division of Vocational Rehabilitation on the agency Appliance Company Referral Form. The DVR Rehabilitation Counselor visited the patient early in the P.T. process and made available his counsel and resources. The following excerpts are from the DVR records:

    June 1   Date of DVR application and financial status report.
    Status 00 Previous family income, $17,000. Expected income,
    Referred $9,800. Client is white, with two-years' college and fifteen years' experience as an accountant. Counselor requested medical reports from the records of the patient's doctors.

June 4 Status 02 Diagnostic	Received general medical report of examination done on April 17.
June 4	Counselor referred patient to the amputee clinic for its next scheduled meeting.
June 9	Patient discharged from hospital and continued the P.T. treatments in extended two-hour daily sessions of exercise and crutch walking. Monthly visits to the doctor.
June 9	DVR preference form signed by client indicating his choice of limb company with which he had been dealing.
June 16	Received narrative surgical history report dictated June 9.
June 18	First amputee clinic visit: "Stump was well-healed, although there was some tenderness over the femoral nerve. It was recommended that patient wear a ladies' long girdle to aid in shrinking of the swollen area, and that he be rechecked at the next amputee clinic in one month." Art didn't like the idea of wearing his wife's girdle, but in a few days saw it was valuable to his sitting comfort and in toughening the scar area. He took exercises and weight lifting at home.
July 16	Second amputee clinic visit: "Ready for fitting. Prescription for a hemipelvectomy prosthesis, the finished prosthesis to be delivered to the amputee clinic." (Arrangements were made with the prosthetist for the client to go to the limb shop on July 20, taking insurance papers with him.)
July 17	Counselor writes to the limb company that insurance will pay 80% of the limb cost.
July 17 Status 10 Accepted	Counselor certified that client was accepted as eligible for DVR services.

July 17
Status 16
Physical
Restoration
Rehabilitation Plan approved by Counselor for the limb cost and gait training and related services above the insurance payment.

July 24 Limb company acknowledges receipt of DVR authorization for full contract price but will bill DVR 20 percent of full cost of limb.

Aug. 5 Mortgage insurance application was denied due to his cancer.

Aug. 7 Wife in office — husband about to crack up. Limb company told him they would not deliver limb until paid for. Counselor cleared with the limb company by phone and called client to reassure him. Client was very eager to get going and get back to work as his sick pay was running out.

Sept. 1 Counselor talked with client's doctor who had wanted client to reenter hospital for his gait training when the limb was delivered. In view of client's feeling of urgency and desire for rapid progress, they agreed that he could bring his prosthesis back with him from the limb company's initial fitting and have it checked immediately by the clinic orthopedist before the next meeting of the amputee clinic scheduled for 16 days later. This out of the ordinary procedure was arranged because of the patient's feeling of great need to spur toward his objective. Out-patient gait training was approved by the doctor since the patient felt he would be more satisfied at home without the irksome confinement of in-patient care. Counselor called the client and advised of the above, and suggested that he call from the limb company if there was any problem regarding delivery of the prosthesis. The client said the company had asked him to give a check for the amount of the prosthesis, and they agreed not to cash it, but would hold it until the insurance money was received by the client.

Sept. 1   Client went to limb company to pick up prosthesis.

Sept. 9   Counselor authorizes special orthopedic examination to check proper fit of limb instead of waiting for the routine checkout at the scheduled amputee clinic time.

Sept. 10 Orthopedic confirming examination done with prescription for 4 to 6 hours P.T. gait training. This was started immediately and continued until the next amputee clinic meeting.

Sept. 17 Third amputee clinic visit: "Walking well in parallel bars and with cane. Continue daily gait training and line the bucket at the limb company shop because of a blister and pressure in sacral area. When the Physical Therapist feels the client can return to work, let the doctor check him and release the limb and the patient can return to work."

The blister held up gait training for a week, but the patient progressed from parallel bars to Canadian crutches and conventional cane. He walked in the hall traffic to the hospital gift shop — then outside — then practiced falling on the mat.

While Art was taking his gait training, the physical therapist arranged for him to meet another patient, a farmer who had the same doctor and who was also scheduled to have a hemipelvectomy amputation. The demonstration of successful achievement that Art represented and described was very valuable to this patient facing such radical surgery, and when Art saw him again later after surgery he was in good spirits. Earlier Art himself had observed a hip disarticulation patient wearing a prosthesis but found that a hemipelvectomy prosthesis is harder to handle in walking and moving. One of Art's office associates also referred an above-knee amputee to him during his hospitalization, for encouragement and advice that were very helpful. The patient saw that Art's problem was more difficult than his, and that it could be conquered. Art also profited from these experiences, as it was good to be told that his visit to the hospital did more for the patient than the visits of all the others combined, except the immediate family, of course. As he met each member of the amputee clinic team, Art felt more confidence because a lot of people were interested in helping him, and he felt he should do his part.

> Oct. 15 Fourth Amputee Clinic visit: "Walking well. A little redness over the sacral area yet, but prosthesis fit satisfactorily and patient is discharged from the Clinic. Recommend return to work half-time as soon as possible, and full-time when he can tolerate the prosthesis for an 8-hour period."

All did not go as smoothly as this terse report indicates. When Art first came in the room, the doctor said "Walk across the room." As the team watched, he said, "Who in Hell taught you to walk? Now walk the other direction," and pushed his limb from behind. The prosthetist said, "Doc, you got more to push with than he has." The counselor asked, "Does he need any more gait training?" and the doctor paused, and finally said, "No." Although the doctor was joking to needle the therapist, the patient didn't realize this and felt hopelessly failing just at the end of his gait training when he thought he had done so well. He did not communicate this deep hurt to the amputee clinic team.

On October 22, Art returned to work half days. He went down to the office the evening before to check the path to his desk, so he wouldn't meet any obstacles that would be awkward when he walked in the first day. All went well, with the help of tranquilizers, and on November 2, he resumed full-time work. His disability pay had been half-pay, so the jump to full-time work was a welcome increase in income. He was allowed an hour and 15 minutes for lunch, so he could lie down and rest at his mother's house which was nearer the office than his own home was. However, later his mother fell and broke her ankle. This was just one in a long list of problems and anxieties over a two-year period affecting his adjustment to his handicap that loomed so large in its impact on the ordinary activities of daily living.

At first everything seemed to be a problem. For example,

1. Sitting without the prosthesis created quite a problem; the prosthesis provided more balance and made sitting more comfortable.

2. Constipation was a problem since some of the elimination muscles were removed in the amputation; but a mild laxative helped.

3. Indigestion was a bother since the prosthesis tends to push into the abdominal wall in sitting, standing and walking.

4. There was worry about financial problems even though the patient had sufficient insurance.

5. The new two-story house appeared to be a big problem, not only financially but in negotiating the stairs; however, with proper training and eventual confidence, climbing the stairway up or down with either crutches or wearing the prosthesis became a routine thing and eventually no problem at all. A hand rail was installed on both sides of the steps, and by using a little foresight and care, no great difficulties were encountered because of the stairs. This training helped when he encountered steps in visiting other homes or in public buildings.

6. People were a problem because some wanted to do everything for the amputee, while others let him try to do the impossible without helping. The amputee was also a problem to himself in that being independent for so many years, he was hesitant to seek or accept help from others when it was really needed.

7. On inclines of more than 10 percent, the knee of the prosthesis would tend to give way. Therefore the amputee had to go down these inclines sideways, being careful to keep the weight of the body ahead of the knee.

8. It took a great deal of physical stamina and exertion to walk even a block since the only muscles available to swing the artificial limb through for a step were the lower abdominal muscles. As a result, speech was also difficult while walking.

9. Walking in a crowd was hazardous since the artificial limb was "Swung through" in taking a step. However, the cane usually alerted the people nearby of the amputee's problem.

10. Almost every activity now took more energy and stamina than before, even sitting. His activities were limited by how much energy he could spend for that activity and the degree of tolerance in time that he could wear the prosthesis. He had to learn to pace himself in this respect. Patience was not one of Art's virtues, and

the frustrations of not being able to do some of the things formerly done led to a more serious problem later.

11. It took a long time to sell his previous house and settle the financial affairs.

12. His office moved and this changed the physical arrangements where he worked.

13. The new house was over-assessed for tax purposes, and protest forms had to be filed and a hearing held.

14. There were difficulties with the Social Security office in obtaining the disability check, which was delayed for almost a year.

15. The couple held their 25th wedding anniversary celebration before he received his prosthesis, and this caused further emotional stress.

16. Four separate school graduations of the children were held in one summer, with the attending strain of arrangements.

17. Being involved in two auto accidents in less than a year, one before and one after the amputation. Art was not driving in one, and not at fault; there were no injuries but considerable damage both times, one a hit-and-run affair.

18. Two daughters were involved in two separate auto accidents, with slight injury to one daughter and total loss of the family car.

19. The necessary purchase of two new autos involved tedious shopping, and return to the dealer for numerous adjustments.

20. Considerable time was spent for all the insurance claims related to the operation, prosthesis and auto accidents.

21. The house mortgage insurance application was denied due to his history of cancer.

22. The insurance company cancelled the auto insurance at Christmas time. Arrangements had to be made for changing companies for further auto coverage.

23. The usual routine problems of a family of nine, one student away at school and six at home.

24. Periodic back sprain of lower back, requiring treatments by an osteopath.

On the positive side, there are many rewards:

1. The first look in the mirror wearing the prosthesis and

trousers. What an improvement over the empty pants leg! Everything else even *looked* better.

2. The first step wearing the prosthesis at the limb company shop, between the parallel bars – a real thrill! And the same thing again a few days later at the hospital.

3. No complications developed in fitting the prosthesis, except the one blister early in the case.

4. Getting behind the wheel of the car and driving a good part of the way on the first trip to the limb company for the fitting – another good feeling.

5. Realizing that a number of activities are possible, with some help in parking:

> Shopping trips, family visits, dinners, picnics.
> Office Christmas parties, luncheons for colleagues.
> Son's Khoury League games.
> Attending childrens' graduations and visiting son at college.
> Going out to dinner with wife and long time friends.
> Bowling, even with a score below 100.
> Fishing, even though the catch is only a little bluegill.
> Yard work, watering the lawn, trimming with shears, sweeping walks, digging, washing car.
> Playing ping pong, if you have help in chasing balls.
> Pitching horse shoes, playing catch with sons.
> Being able to help around the house: run vacuum cleaner, dishwasher, make beds, dusting, sweeping, washing, preparing foods for the freezer and even painting halfway up on a stepladder.

Continuing DVR records show the following:

Oct. 23   Acceptance form signed by client that the prosthesis is satisfactory. No additional comments were given.

Oct. 23   Letter from client to counselor: "Dear Joe, Just a note to thank you for your time and effort spent on my behalf. I certainly appreciated it as did my wife. I started working half days this week and when I can stand it (to wear the prosthesis all day) will resume full-time work (I hope) in a week or two. Thanks again. Sincerely, Art Craig."

Dec. 8	Client returned employment information inquiry form showing his employer, address, date he returned to work Oct. 22, as an accountant at $200 per week. No additional comments were given in the space provided for comments or suggestions.
Dec. 14	Counselor canceled authorization to hospital for unused out-patient visits. A total of 22 were used. Case ready for closure.
Jan. 8 Status 26 Closed Rehab	Counselor closed case records and wrote a letter to client informing him of this action, with a carbon to the limb company who was the referral source.

On December 18, unknown to DVR, the client wrote a letter to his congressman asking his help after 5 months' wait in getting a reply from the VA acknowledging his claim for service connection of his cancer to his 9 months' prisoner of war status in WWII with inhumane treatment, poor diet and various deprivations following his capture after a parachute jump severely spraining his leg. He stated,

> "Since no one knows what causes cancer, how could anyone definitely say this is non-service connected? Therefore, I believe I am entitled to some kind of pension — I don't know how long I will be able to work full-time (I returned on Nov. 1, 1960)."

On January 5, the client received a VA letter of denial and forwarded it to his congressman. The findings were subsequently appealed twice but denied both times.

Meanwhile, Art continued to work full-time for 5 months at his job which was sedentary. At the time of his second auto accident he took sick leave for one month and ten days, and then returned to work regularly, missing only three days in the next ten months. His employer was very considerate, but his work sometimes required him to travel and attend meetings both away and in his home town. All of his problems mentioned previously were weighing on him, and he worried especially about an impending business trip that would be too exhausting by auto, so he planned to go by small plane. This caused access problems, and the exertion of the new experience aggravated him. Overnight in a motel, he needed a walker like he used at home but he didn't have one. He took a sleeping pill to calm down and get some rest, but when he got up he was groggy and fell, hurting his side, but most of all his pride. It was discouraging. "Is this all I can do," he thought, "can't manage a simple trip?" He felt his faith was severely tested to answer the question, "Why?, and Why me?"

He tried to carry on as he did before, but the exertion, the frustrations and anxiety were too much for him. On March 22, a year and a half after return to work he collapsed and took sick leave under the recommendation and care of a new doctor, a general physician, who wrote, in a report for Social Security disability benefits,

> Mr. Craig is prostrated by nervous exhaustion. This is a result of the valiant effort he made in adjusting physically and emotionally to wearing the prosthesis with which he was fitted after his surgery. He was determined to return to work walking and without needing anyone's assistance, as soon as possible. He pushed too hard and is now on an extended leave of absence from his job, and may be able to return to it eventually.

He did go to church on Easter and wore the prosthesis for one hour and returned home to bed. He was up and down irregularly till May 1, when he started to wear the prosthesis more. By June 1 he could wear the limb 8 to 10 hours at a time, and attended a Memorial Day picnic. However, he tended to stay away from crowds.

June 8 he received his Social Security disability benefits award, and by mid-July could wear the limb 12 hours at a time. He then planned a family vacation, and traveled in the mountains before his return to work in September.

Art Craig's primary concern during the rehabilitation process was to prepare for a life as near to his former life style as possible under the circumstances: a return to the home and the everyday task of living, a return to the job and its responsibilities and duties and a continuation of his spiritual life and recreational and social activities. In pressing so hard to reach these objectives so perfectly, completely and quickly, he nearly lost the considerable achievement he had already accomplished up to then.

A conspicuous deficit in the casework was the omission of psychological evaluation or social casework study. It is axiomatic in rehabilitation that if a client has substantial problems in any one of medical, psychological, social or vocational areas, he is sure to have problems in the other three areas. No vocational tests were needed; he had 15 years' experience and his old job was waiting for him when he was ready. The team tried to meet his needs in making exceptions to the usual routine because they recognized the urgency the patient felt in straining toward his goals. But no formal personality assessment was made nor personal, psychological counseling done; and this turned out to be the biggest problem that nearly wrecked the good work done in overcoming the physical problems. A social worker's evaluation would have spotlighted the patient's extreme drive and motivation of a "good" client and cautioned the rehabilitation team that this might be a danger as well as an asset.

The client concluded,

> As the days, months and years go by, there will be even more changes, accidents and frustrations to cope with. Rehabilitation is a continuing process even on my own. But it sure beats being dead.

DISCUSSION QUESTIONS

1. Discuss types of cancer in relation to disabling characteristics (Hodgkins Disease, Leukemia, Carcinoma, Melanomia, Sarcoma).
2. Discuss vocational environments which should be avoided in special cases.

SUGGESTED READING

Cancer Facts and Figures, American Cancer Society, 1970.

Cutler, S. James and Heise, H.W. Long-term End Results of Treatment of Cancer. JAMA, 216:293, 1971.

Hardy, R.E. and Cull, J.G. Counseling and Rehabilitating the Cancer Patient, Springfield: Charles C Thomas, 1974.

Hardy, R.E. and Cull, J.G. Severe Disabilities: Social and Rehabilitation Approaches. Springfield, Thomas, 1973.

Healey, J.E., Jr. Changing Philosophy Toward Rehabilitation. Cancer Bull, 20:2-3, January-February, 1968.

Holleb, A.I. Using the Cancer Cures We have Now. Today's Health, April, 1970.

Kelly, William D. and Friesen, Staley R. Do Cancer Patients want to be told? Surgery, 27:822-26, 1950.

Knudson, Alfred G., Jr. Genetics and Cancer. Postgrad Med, Vol. 48, No. 5, November, 1970.

Li, Frederick P. et al Familial Ovarian Carcinoma. Journal of the American Medical Association, 214, 1970.

Mayer, J. Nutrition and Cancer, Part I. Postgraduate Medicine, 50, 1971.

Mayer, J. Nutrition and Cancer, Part II Postgraduate Medicine, 50, 1971.

Mozden, Peter J., Neoplasms. In Julian S. Myers (Ed.) An Orientation to Chronic Disease and Disability. New York, The MacMillan Company, 1965, p. 323.

Rehabilitation Record, Vol. 7, No. 1, January-February, 1966.

Research Brief of Significant Findings–Rehabilitation of Cancer Patients, Memorial Hospital for Cancer and Allied Diseases, New York, New York.

Rusk, H.A. Preventive Medicine, Curative Medicine – The Rehabilitation. New Physician, 13:5-167, 1964.

Skimkin, Michael B. Duration of life on untreated cancer. Cancer, 4:1, 1951.

Teaching About Cancer. Publication of the American Cancer Society.

Wargensteen, Owen H. Should patients be told they have cancer, (Ed.). Surgery, 27:944-947, 1950.

Youth Looks at Cancer. American Cancer Society.

Chapter 11

DEAFNESS AND ITS EFFECTS

Attitudes Toward Deafness
Reasons for Attitudes
Facts Reguarding Deafness
Employer – Employee Relations
Adjustment Problems on the Job
Facts About California Department of Rehabilitation's Program
Case Studies
Discussion Questions
Suggested Reading

ATTITUDES TOWARD DEAFNESS

WHEN I started to work with deaf and hard-of-hearing persons in 1967, I had no idea of the extent of their exclusion from society. After a short time it became clear that they were given second-class citizenship. They were shortchanged in education, ignored or downgraded in employment, tolerated in society and often buffooned in the theatre. They were looked upon, in general, as not only without hearing, but without mind; deaf and dumb. All of the language I had heard for years came into focus, such as when children do not respond, "Are you deaf and dumb?", or "Hey, dummy" or "What's the matter, stupid? Can't you hear?" So these notions kept deaf persons a group apart from the hearing world. They were forced to form their own segregated groups where they could not only be understood, but could find refuge from the stares, often condescending, of hearing persons.

I was and am distressed to observe that not only do hearing nonprofessionals stereotype deaf persons as a group, but so do the professional workers. I am aware that we all shortout communication. However, it seems strange to me that among professionals, working in the field of deafness, hearing handicapped persons are lumped together as "the deaf," "the hard of hearing." Although persons with hearing loss, total or partial, are all individuals, they are viewed, at least in the term describing them, as a type or species. This terminology, it seems to me, removes their individual differences and highlights only their sameness. As I see it, disabled persons, regardless of their medical condition are persons who happen to have some physical, mental or emotional deviation which causes them particular problems. To me, it is a mistake to speak of "the deaf," "the hard-of-hearing," "the blind," "the mentally retarded," etc. As I stated previously, I am sure this is all done for quick identification, but I think it identifies and reinforces the weaknesses instead of the strengths.

What is inherent in the physical disability and what is caused by other factors? Mentally retarded persons are the way they are because of certain inherent limitations of their intellectual capacities. They are able to achieve up to a limited level only. There is a ceiling on the amount of information they can assimilate. The mental condition itself, therefore, is the handicap.

With blind persons we have learned that the absence or limitation of vision, in and of itself, does not have within it barriers to learning and training for work. It has been shown, over and over again, that with proper training, first mobility, then educational or vocational, blind persons can become functioning and contributing members of society. It has been demonstrated that they can achieve high goals and that there is a wide range of ability, just as there is in the general population.

REASONS FOR ATTITUDES

Little by little, progress is being made in the understanding about deaf persons. There is little inherent in the disability that creates the problems. It is the lack of services because of our lack of understanding that creates the problems.

There are some basic principles of human behavior that are pertinent to attitudes toward hearing handicapped persons. When we address someone, we expect a response. If no response is forthcoming, we make several assumptions: 1) he is ignoring us; this infuriates us; 2) he does not understand us; this makes us uncomfortable and anxious. The methods we have of handling our own feelings are: 1) to get even, 2) to relieve our own anxiety by leaving the scene. It never occurs to most of us that perhaps the person may just not have been able to hear us. Maybe his language understanding does not include the words we have employed.

An interesting commentary is that if we were traveling in a foreign country and spoke to a native, we would: 1) try to learn something of his language, 2) repeat in a way he might understand, perhaps by gesture, 3) look for an interpreter.

Until now the above has not applied to our contacts with deaf persons. We have avoided them, whenever possible. If we have been unable to avoid them, as in professional contacts, we have done whatever had been the easiest, avoided communication. We have categorized them as uninterested or nonmotivated if they have objected to our techniques. Those who are compliant are placed in jobs far beneath their capacities.

There is a basic difference between deaf persons and foreigners. In a foreign country, the visitor is the stranger and he must make the effort to be understood. Also, it is quite obvious that there is a language barrier. Deafness does not show. The person looks like everyone else. In our verbal society, we judge people by what they say. We often give meaning to what we hear beyond the actual words themselves. We interpret noises we hear in light of our moods or our moods are created by the sounds we hear. Our listeners respond to what we say by doing certain things, responding to our speech in like manner or making certain facial expressions.

A person with a hearing loss is denied this kind of interchange. He cannot hear the words; therefore, he cannot respond in the expected fashion, whether it be to do what is requested or to answer a question. He is unable even to make the appropriate facial grimades. He is, in essence, looking at a blank wall and responding to it, in kind, blankly. He may defend his inadequacy by smiling because he knows a smile is a sure indicator of friendliness. The conversation may not intend to elicit a smile; this is unknown to him. His smile, he hopes, will satisfy the speaker in some way. It serves often only to categorize him as "stupid."

Because deafness is invisible to all intents and purposes, it does not exist. The human tendency is to avert one's eyes from something one wants to avoid. This is not necessary in dealing with deaf persons. We do not have to use the mechanism "out of sight – out of mind." If the individual is hard-of-hearing and wearing a hearing aid, we know something is the matter, but in our mechanistic orientation, it seems only necessary to turn it on or up, and everything will be OK.

Many hearing-handicapped persons themselves reinforce the view of the hearing population. They depend upon lip reading for understanding. It has been estimated that only 23 percent of the population can learn to speechread effectively. Those few manage to get along. The others guess at what is said and though they feel they are part of the hearing world, they are not. There are several ways deaf people see and group themselves. They either try to align themselves with the hearing population, and by refusing to use manual communication, they think they are part of the hearing population. They may go to the other extreme and associate only with other deaf persons. They can accept themselves as deaf or hard-of-hearing, thereby, gaining status in their own groups and also having a place in hearing groups. The latter approach has to be a two-way interaction. It is not possible as long as suspicion and disrespect are present.

All of the above shows how little understanding exists about deafness. There is disagreement even among experts about the thinking processes of deaf people. For some time, the opinion was that all deaf persons were intellectually slower than hearing persons. This was based on the results of verbal tests validated on hearing persons with language. Furthermore, these tests were administered by testers who had no experience in testing deaf persons. Also the tests were group tests and not suitable for deaf persons who need to be tested individually, or at least given individual instructions. Myklebust and Levine, psychologists with experience in dealing with deaf persons, tried nonverbal material and reached the conclusion that when suitable test instruments were used in suitable conditions, "deaf persons displayed the same range of abilities as everyone else." At Oregon State School for the Deaf, it was demonstrated by Dr. Bannich that when each student was tested nonverbally, there was the same range of differences as among hearing people. Hans Furth, Catholic University, Washington, D.C. came up with the same conclusion. The consensus was that deaf persons were like everyone else except they had communication problems.

FACTS REGARDING DEAFNESS

Ever so gradually, there has been developing an interest and concern for that part of our population with hearing disabilities. It has been necessary to define deafness and to consider the age of onset. The age of onset is important to begin assessment of individual's development of language. We need to know the kind of hearing impairment, the nature and extent of other organic defects, the environment in which the individual lives and his education.

To begin to assess deaf children's aptitudes and interests, work and thought is being given to identification of suitable instruments. Some of the prevailing instruments were found useful for typical groups in specific ways. To be valid for a deaf child, the instrument must be nonverbal, for there has been no development of speech and language or there has been little increase in language understanding, and verbal tests are not fair or valid. Verbal tests with deaf children measure language deficiency due to hearing loss rather than measuring intelligence. There have been innumerable cases of people whose major problem is deafness being sent to institutions for retarded persons on the basis of low test scores. Even some nonverbal tests are not appropriate because they require verbal directions. Hard-of-hearing children may give the impression of being able to understand verbal tests, but this is often an artifice. It is advisable to begin these children with a performance test and then, if desired, a verbal instrument may be tried. In cases where the performance score is appreciably higher, the probability is that the lower score on the test involving language is due to hearing impairment and does not constitute a true measure of intelligence.

EMPLOYER – EMPLOYEE RELATIONS

The employer group, as a whole, has had little contact with deaf persons. This is due to the communication barrier and the time consumption of using writing for transmission of information. Employers need to be convinced that people can learn by written message and by demonstration. One of the best means of convincing them is to point out the employment record of hearing-handicapped workers. It may be worth it to an employer to avoid excessive and expensive turnover by spending extra time training a deaf worker who will be a responsible and loyal employee. It is up to the schools for deaf children and special education programs to teach about job responsibility and loyalty.

The general problems a deaf person faces when he applies for work are many. They are the immediate communication lack, the employer's long standing attitudes regarding deafness created by past experiences with deaf persons and by prejudice, lack of social understanding and the technical ability.

As all workers, a deaf worker's continued employment and job advancement depend on his ability to perform his entry job well and to respond to training. Unlike others, however, he has the additional obligation to develop a means of communication with his shop boss and fellow workers.

Educators of deaf children need to emphasize employee roles and responsibilities, and to acquaint them with the world as it is, not as it looks.

Even a trained, well-adjusted deaf person runs into stumbling blocks. Unprepared and inexperienced deaf job seekers have even more difficulty. The vocational programs in schools for the deaf are not complete or up-to-date. The graduate goes out into the labor market poorly prepared, educationally retarded and socially inept.

He may try to apply for work accompanied by a hearing individual. Sometimes this serves only to raise questions about his "self-sufficiency." His inability to fill out application forms reinforces notions that he is mentally slow. His inability to read and interpret test instructions will handicap him in taking written job knowledge or aptitude and intelligence tests. The job interview, itself, will be an obstacle.

Lack of skill in applying for a job, deficiency in entry work skills, inadequate written language, lack of functional oral language all serve to bar a deaf applicant from employment. Job hunting techniques need to be taught in schools for the deaf and special education programs for the hearing handicapped. How to dress, how to present one's self to a receptionist, how to complete an application, how to write a resume and how to present it are all facets of securing employment.

The job resume needs to include an initial statement explaining the individual is deaf and is seeking work. If he lipreads, he should indicate this and explain the suitable conditions to accomplish this. This should be followed by personal data, educational and vocational training, work experience, hobbies and interests. This should be taught as a supplement to vocational training.

Also, schools need to expose graduates to personnel, aptitude and job knowledge tests and to acquaint them with test-taking techniques.

The students could also be given experience in interviewing prospective employers by role-playing sessions in school. The stumbling blocks in job hunting are known. We need to prepare students for them.

ADJUSTMENT PROBLEMS ON THE JOB

After an individual is placed, adjustment problems may become evident. For deaf persons, these are often more extreme because of the communication barrier. The lack of understanding and knowledge about job loyalty and responsibility are barriers to continued employment and promotion. These need to be explored and explained as part of the vocational training program. Teaching skills is not enough. Work attitudes are equally important. Good work attitudes often are more important than great skill. An employer will often overlook an individual's lack of skill, if he likes the individual. He may even take time to teach him in order to retain him in the organization.

The greatest single problem on the job does not seem to be the deaf person's acquisition of job skills. It hinges, rather, on his erratic work habits and, often, anti-social behavior. Schools need to enlarge their curricula to include courses on responsibility of an employee to an employer. There needs to be increased communication between schools and employers.

We define rehabilitation as the "restoration of an individual to the maximum level of social, emotional and vocational functioning of which he is capable." In the case of many deaf persons, it is "habilitation" because they are not to be "restored" but "started" on the way toward functioning. For those who are hard-of-hearing, this is also true, for many of them have never been given the opportunity to exercise their maximum functioning. Instead of their ability, it has been their disability that has been emphasized. Unlike the popular song, we have "exaggerated the negative and eliminated the positive."

The progress that is being made by hearing-handicapped persons aided by hearing individuals is encouraging. Deaf workers, in general, have a good record. Their counterparts among hearing persons leave jobs because they want a "voice" in the management. A "foot in the door" is what deaf people want. The door is gradually being pushed open. Hopefully, deaf persons will be allowed to get to the top floor.

FACTS ABOUT CALIFORNIA DEPARTMENT OF REHABILITATION'S PROGRAM

The California Department of Rehabilitation became concerned over its lack of personnel able to communicate with deaf persons. For some time there were only two counselors for deaf persons, one in Northern California and one in Southern California. In 1963 the Department, newly formed under its own director, began an active program to assign counselors to specialize with hearing-handicapped persons. These counselors were provided with training in sign-language and courses related to the psychology of deafness and special problems encountered by deaf persons.

These counselors received all of the deaf and hard-of-hearing applicants and built up a case-load of these persons. It was interesting to observe that many deaf persons had previously been denied services on the basis they were employed and, therefore, had no vocational handicap. When they saw a counselor who understood them, could communicate with them and who realized that they were definitely underemployed, their cases were reopened and necessary training provided for more suitable occupations. The counselors for deaf and hard-of-hearing persons embarked upon a community education program enlightening as many persons as possible to the abilities of deaf people. The counselors also learned more about their own communities, becoming acquainted with hearing persons involved with deaf persons and able to communicate with them. Thus, people who could be used as interpreters, tutors and aides were found. The counselors also learned about social, church and educational resources for their clients. Not only did deaf persons benefit, but so did the counselors whose horizons had expanded.

Currently there are special counselors for hearing-handicapped persons in each rehabilitation district of the state. Some of them have secretaries and aides who know sign-language. There is also a full-time coordinator of services to deaf persons on the central office staff.

CASE STUDIES

The following are case studies from my case load. Some individuals have achieved and some have not. The reasons are not clear but good family relationships seem to contribute to individuals' feelings of self-worth.

Case A

In 1969, a short, poorly dressed and ill-kempt man of 33 appeared at the Los Angeles office of the Department of Rehabilitation writing down "I am deaf — need job and money." He indicated he had a place to stay, was vague about where he'd come from but insisted he would work if he had suitable training. He was referred to the counselor for the deaf who communicated in sign-language. She determined he had gone to a school for the deaf to the tenth grade and had quit. He reported he was divorced and his wife had custody of their child who was six years old at that time. He asked for training in body and fender repair and seemed motivated, so was enrolled in a trade school in Los Angeles. He gave every indication of having been a floater but seemed interested in settling down.

He was referred to welfare by the vocational rehabilitation counselor and he was housed in the unattached men's service center. Because the welfare process was slow, vocational rehabilitation provided maintenance and transportation as well as training fees and purchased tools for him during training. The training plan was to be of twenty-eight weeks duration at a cost of: $1,090.00

Tools	410.22
Transportation	117.04
Maintenance	475.00
Total	$2,092.26

The week he started, he missed several days due to abdominal complaints. He returned after a few days and then missed again, reporting he'd been involved in an auto accident. He did not return to school and in the meantime, the school closed up and it became necessary to secure another training resource. The rehabilitation counselor took him to various shops to try to analyze on-the-job training. A shop was located which agreed to pay a wage to him as a regular employee. He requested and was given additional tools from the agency stockroom and others were purchased amounting to $149. He accepted all the tools but worked only one week saying he's been laid off because he had a back problem and was unable to do the work. He kept the tools saying he expected to return to work when his condition improved. He did not return to work. Instead he applied for welfare insisting still that this was temporary. A month later he was hired by a body and fender man who knew sign-language. He was arrested the next day for begging on the street. The employer still decided to take him back, however.

A week later the man was fired because of excessive absences and drinking on the job. He was picked up for vagrancy several times. Efforts were made to get our tools back, but it was learned the man had moved, leaving no forwarding address.

He returned sometime later saying he'd been ill and in need of hospitalization. He also spoke of a possible job where he would use the tools. Instead of going to work he went to jail for vagrancy. While in jail, he wrote the name of his rehabilitation counselor and she was called to the Women's Probation Department where the man was being held for impersonation.

He then disappeared with the tools and a year later appeared at the Sacramento, California, office. Efforts were made to get the tools back but the man reported they'd been stolen. He asked for more tools but was told none would be issued until he secured work which could be verified.

Because of his poor past record I couldn't recommend him to employers. He receives Aid to the Disabled of $140 per month. He keeps saying he wants a job but it is questionable he will get one.

Medical Information This man has a severe congenital bilateral sensori-neural hearing loss. Only speech awareness thresholds could be established since he could distinguish no test words. A hearing aid was purchased for him as one seemed helpful but he never wore it.

Case B

Mr. B., an engineer, and his wife, who is a college graduate and whose main goal in life was to be a mother and wife, enjoyed their two lovely blonde children, a girl and boy, three years apart in age. Mrs. B. spent all of her time with them, making up games and songs and enjoying their wide-eyed appreciation. Their playmates were involved with them and the B.'s home was the "fun-place" of the block.

In 1950 when the little girl was three, the family decided to spend Thanksgiving in Los Angeles with good friends. The little girl's birthday was to be celebrated that same week. Preparations for the trip were made excitedly and in great anticipation. The day before departure the little girl suddenly complained of a very sore nape of the neck. The family pediatrician was called and he ordered a spinal tap. This test was negative but the child's fever zoomed and she went into a coma. She was immediately hospitalized and a diagnosis of influenzal meningitis was made. Medication was instantly prescribed. The child was in a coma about three days and in the hospital, nineteen. As soon as she came out of the coma, her mother realized the child had lost her hearing. She also had no balance and could not walk. She was extremely fearful and clung to her mother and father when they visited. The mother was permitted to be with her constantly.

When the child came home, her parents devoted all of their time to her. They gave up their social activities, played with her constantly and were with her through her waking hours and sat near her until they were sure she was fast asleep.

The mother continued her activities and spoke to the child as she had before, using familiar words and introducing new ones as the situation demanded them. The child had always been precocious and had spoken early so she had a considerable vocabulary to start with.

The child's walking ability did not return for one year and it took about one and one-half years for her to regain her confidence in herself and her trust in others. The parents took her to a speech and hearing clinic to try to learn how to communicate better with her. While there, they learned of the John Tracy Clinic in Southern California and its program to teach lip-reading to hearing-impaired persons.

The family applied and was accepted for the summer program. The mother and two children stayed for six weeks. The father was able to come only during his two-weeks vacation period. The family learned about speech reading and the child's trust and self-confidence increased. The rest of the family became more confident and lost some of their helpless feeling. Their pattern of doing things together continued. There had never been any recrimination about the situation, as all that could be done had been done. The parents were extremely supportive of each other, as they had always been. The children received as much attention, if not more, as they always had. The little boy was not neglected. He was involved in a family situation and was a very important factor in it.

When the child was four a special class was set up in a school away from her neighborhood in which there were three other deaf children. The child was accepted as a five-year-old as she was advanced for her age. At about this same time the parents discussed the mother's eligibility for a teaching credential and made plans for her to secure it. She had demonstrated her ability by working with her own and other deaf children as she had volunteered in the special class. She realized her responsibility to deaf children but before going ahead for a credential she and her husband discussed the unsuitability of their child being in a school away from her neighborhood and friends. They were able, therefore, to have her accepted in the neighborhood school where she went one hour each morning, after going to the other school. She stayed in neighborhood schools throughout her school years, never going to special classes. She was graduated from a regular high school where she made excellent grades. She wore binaural hearing aids which brought in no speech but only sounds. She sat in front where she could read the teachers' lips and was well adjusted.

She had many friends and became a junior hospital volunteer, a Peppermint. She soon was president of that organization. In that position she had to do a great deal of telephone communication. Her parents had heard of a special telephone in which the earphone and the mouthpiece are separate. They secured one and when the phone rang, the mother listened to the message, spoke it to the girl who gave the answer herself. She, therefore, used her voice all the time and preserved its quality. Part of her job was to be involved with the children's hospital and her colleagues as well as her mother assisted with the telephone procedure.

Because of her hospital involvement she became interested in nursing and selected a small Catholic college in San Francisco to attend. Her parents realized she could not be a nurse without a hearing associate always at her side, but the girl insisted. Before she started to college, however, the head of nursing confirmed the parents' advice and the girl changed to journalism and later to an English major. The Department of Rehabilitation underwrote her college plan, though ordinarily private colleges are not used. The family had made such an intensive study of the value of a small intimate college to the girl, however, that it was allowed. The agency paid also for notetaker services to allow other students to take and go over notes for the girl. She, herself, in her self-assured way talked to the instructors many of whom loaned her their own notes to study or gave her additional work material. She secured her B.A. in June 1971.

In the meantime at a girl friend's house she met a young man and fell in love. She decided to get whatever work she could and live at home to save money. She secured work as a clerk-typist for the state and is saving her money toward marriage. Her fiance is in the service and hopes to go to school upon discharge.

Her mother, in the meantime has become an expert on speechreading and is a consultant in the field of cued speech for the school district. She works full-time as an elementary school teacher.

The family relationship is a close one with all members being respected and well-regarded. The girl's accomplishments are due greatly to this as well as to her native ability.

Case C

Mr. and Mrs. G. had been married for twenty years without having children. Mrs. G. then conceived and with great joy produced a son. He was handsome and cheerful but somehow, unresponsive. It was not until he was two that his deafness was revealed. Up until that point he had been viewed as a slow learner. His parents kept him in the house fearful that he would get hurt. He had no friends and spent time only in the house. He had no speech. His mother mouthed to him and pointed out what she meant but he did not learn to lip read; he only followed her motions and actions.

When it was time for him to go to school his parents tentatively enrolled him at the California School for the Deaf in Berkeley, California. They allowed him to stay a very short time as they "worried about him" and brought him home. He was enrolled in day school but could not get along and there were no aurally handicapped classes at that time. John then stayed at home playing alone or with his mother.

When he was twenty-one he went to work as a laborer in a mattress factory at a very low wage. He then went to work as a laborer in a smoke house leaving that for another labor job. He worked at labor until 1951 when his parents bought a motel in Idaho and he worked as janitor and yardman. His parents stayed in the motel business until they retired in 1969 and John helped them.

John was committed to a state mental institution in 1956, when he developed a chronic drinking problem and became hostile and difficult to manage. He was discharged in 1957 to his parents and stayed at home for the next two years. In 1959 he was recommitted with a diagnosis of sociopathic personality disturbance and alcoholism. He remained in the hospital one year and again returned home. He was recommitted one year later remaining in the hospital for two years then placed on day care under supervision of his parents. He was discharged from the hospital three years later and referred to a psychiatric social worker who referred him to vocational rehabilitation.

At our first contact, John used rudimentary sign language, mostly home-made signs. His mother seemed distressed that she was left out of the conversation. She kept interjecting her own conversational technique of mouthing and pointing. It was very apparent that John needed association with other deaf people. I asked a deaf man to visit him and interest him in coming to the deaf club. John's mother discouraged this. Though she did not say so, her concern seemed to be related to her fear of her son's drinking problem. His behavior since his discharge from the hospital has been good but he has been at home all of the time and watched by her. She spoke of electronic assembly as a good field for him as he had good manual dexterity. I learned that the San Jose' Goodwill had contracts from Lockheed and was doing training in electronic assembly. John's mother who did all of the negotiating for him felt this would be a good spot for him. They were given a transportation allowance and the mother drove them to San Jose. John has no driver's license because of his drinking history. When they returned, the mother and John expressed satisfaction with the training but decided against moving to San Jose as John's father was ailing and getting worse. The mother decided nothing should be done at that time and we closed our case.

Two years later the mother reapplied for help for her son. He had been struck by a hit-and-run driver and was in the hospital with mangled legs and there was some question of his mobility upon recovery. He also had a badly lacerated face and was scheduled for plastic surgery.

The parents were still operating a motel and their concern was about John's employability upon recovery. He had been helping around the motel but this would no longer be possible if his legs did not improve. It took six months for his casts to be removed and six more months for him to be out of a wheelchair. The mother insisted on our maintaining contact throughout this period and when John was out of the wheelchair he and his mother asked for training. I was willing to arrange a prevocational program but transportation presented a problem. The mother refused to allow John to get a driver's license and she could not transport him daily so again we closed our case.

Two years later the mother reapplied saying she and her husband had retired from the motel business and John needed work. Efforts were made to locate employment to no avail. The mother then decided to make some contacts of her own and the case was closed. Two years later the mother reapplied reporting her husband had died and she and her son were trying to adjust to this. The family income was Social Security for the mother, Social Security Disability and Aid to the Disabled for the son. He had been drawing this aid throughout our contact. The mother has become even more involved with him and though she speaks of worrying about his future, she places obstacles in the road of planning. By this time John is 51, has little communication ability and is a very dependent person. Unless we can secure work for him as a laborer, which he has done where communication is minimal we again will have to close his case. This is an example of a situation in which social services were required long ago to prepare this family for releasing John and allowing him to grow up.

Case D

Mr. W. a law student married a secretary who worked to help put him through law school. After graduation from law school and just before he entered practice they decided to have children. Their first daughter was beautiful and responsive. Their second daughter was beautiful and nonresponsive and it was discovered she was congenitally deaf due to rubella that the mother suffered early in pregnancy. The parents spent time with their children, spoke to them both as if they could hear and were not hesitant about taking their deaf child with them wherever they went.

The marriage split up, however, due to incompatibility and the father remarried. The mother took in boarders so she could stay home with her children. As they grew up they helped her with the cleaning and cooking. The mother opened a board and care facility and the girls had much company.

The little deaf girl went to regular classes. She was well behaved and quiet and was ignored in class as "she was no trouble." She then was placed in the aurally-handicapped class in high school. She did unusually well, so well in fact that the question arose about the validity of her hearing loss. Otological exams confirmed a profound bilateral sensori-neural hearing loss with not enough residual hearing to conduct a speech discrimination test. She was, however, able to discriminate speech with visual clues. She had worn a hearing aid since early childhood.

She had no useable speech, knew no sign language and was a poor lip-reader. She had fair command of language and could write understandably.

She was not referred to Department of Rehabilitation immediately from high school because of lack of interest. She came in on her own, however, a year later. She was sent to a local business college for a key-punch training course. Upon completion a job was secured for her in San Francisco. She stayed six months and returned to Sacramento because she was lonely. Another job was found for her with the federal government. She did very well and began to mix with deaf people. She also learned sign language. She asked for and was given a tranfer to Washington, D.C. so she could attend classes at Gallaudet College. She is taking classes and working and was named federal employee of the year at one time.

Case E

Robert is twenty-five. He has five hearing siblings and one deaf sister, Helene. He lost his hearing when he was two as a result of a high fever accompanying a case of the mumps. He had just started talking a great deal when he lost his hearing. The shock of his inability to hear was great on his parents but didn't seem to disturb his siblings and friends who continued to play with him and who soon developed a means of communication. His parents, too, after their initial shock developed a means of communication.

Two years later a baby girl was born deaf. The reason was never determined. The mother, having one deafened child and having had time to get used to this, did not feel too shocked, mainly startled. All of the children spent time with the baby enjoying her cuddliness and beauty. She learned to understand them. She, too, as she grew older, played with the neighborhood children.

Robert started school in his home community in a class for hearing-handicapped children. This class was one morning per week. He was transferred to the California School for the Deaf in Berkeley at age seven and went there through high school. His sister started there at age five and went to the tenth grade dropping out to marry a classmate. She completed high school and secured her diploma from a home teacher after several years. Her husband who was a dropout from the School for the Deaf also completed his high school education after several years.

Robert upon graduation was referred to the Department of Rehabilitation counselor in his home district. He is an alert, pleasant, eager young man and at first was placed in a training program in an offset printing establishment. He had been in the print shop at the school. He did well, but the firm went out of business. He then was placed with several other deaf persons in a letter-sorting position at the post-office. Training was required first and an interpreter was paid to help in the training. Robert has been working over two years and is earning over $3 per hour. He was married two years ago to a colleague from the School for the Deaf and she is a keypunch operator for the state.

Helene's husband secured work in electronic assembly but he left the job and she and he moved to Sacramento to be near her family. They asked for help from the Department of Rehabilitation. Helene wanted training in typing and keypunch. She was sent to business college but upon completion we could not find a job for her in keypunch. Since she was a good seamstress and expressed interest in getting a job doing sewing, a job was secured for her in this field. After she worked six months at sewing, a keypunch job was secured for her in the office where her sister-in-law works.

Her husband completed auto-mechanic training under rehabilitation sponsorship and we are now in the process of seeking work for him.

DISCUSSION QUESTIONS

1. Discuss the "deaf personality": Does it exist? If so, what is it?
2. Discuss vocational environments which should be avoided by deaf persons.
3. Discuss the effects of sudden loss of hearing and gradual loss of hearing.
4. What are the types of special diagnostic information needed for vocational planning?
5. Discuss immediate availability of rehabilitation services as a factor in adjustment.
6. Discuss age of onset as a factor in adjustment to hearing loss and total deafness.

SUGGESTED READING

Babbidge, H.D. (Ed.). Education of the Deaf; A report to the Secretary of Health, Education, and Welfare by his advisory committee on the education of the deaf. Washington, D.C., U.S. Department of Health, Education, and Welfare, 1965.

Best, H. Deafness and the Deaf in the United States. New York, MacMillan, 1943.

Crammatte, A.B., (Ed.) Proceedings of the Workshop on Communication Development Through Organizations of and for the Deaf. Washington, D.C., Office of Vocational Rehabilitation, Government Printing Office, 1961.

Furth, H.G. Thinking Without Language: Psychological Implications of Deafness. New York, The Free Press, 1966.

Hardy, R.E. and Cull, J.G. Psychosocial and Educational Aspects of Deafness. Springfield, Thomas, 1974.

Hardy, R.E. and Cull, J.G. Severe Disabilities: Social and Rehabilitation Approaches. Springfield, Thomas, 1973.

Kohl, H.R. Language and education of the deaf. Center for Urban Education, 1966, No. 1.

Kronenberg, H.H. and Blake, G.D. Young deaf adults; An occupational survey. Washington, D.C., Vocational Rehabilitation Administration, U.S. Department of Health, Education, and Welfare, 1966.

Levine, E.S. The Psychology of Deafness. New York, Columbia University Press, 1960.

Lloyd, T.T. (Ed.) International Research Seminar on the Vocational Rehabilitation of Deaf Persons. Washington, D.C., Social and Rehabilitation Service, U.S. Department of H.E.W., 1968.

Lunde, A.S. and Bigman, S.K. Occupational Conditions Among the Deaf. Washington, D.C., Gallaudet College, 1959.

MacKane, K. A Comparison of the Intelligence of Deaf and Hearing Children. New York, Columbia University, 1933.

Mayes, T.A. Education and rehabilitation of the deaf: A candid view. Deaf Am, 22:9-11, 1970.

Myklebust, H.R. The Psychology of Deafness. New York, Grune and Stratton, 1960.

Newman, L. The handicap of deafness, Deaf Am, 24:18, 1972.

Ranier, J.D. and Altschuler, K.Z. Comprehensive Mental Health Services for the Deaf. New York, Department of Medical Genetics, New York Psychiatric Institute, 1966.

Ranier, J.D., Altschuler, K.Z., Kallman, F.J., and Deming, W.E., Family and mental health problems in a deaf population. New York, Columbia University, 1963.

Stuckless, E.R. and Birch, J.M. The influence of early manual communication on the linguistic development of deaf children. Am Ann Deaf, 111:452-62, 1966.

Switzer, M.E. and Williams, B.R. Life problems of deaf people. Arch Environ Health, 15:249-256, 1967.

Vernon, M. Mental health, deafness and communication. In D.M. Denton (Ed.), Proceedings of the teachers institute. Frederick, Md., Maryland School for the Deaf, 1969, pp. 16-18.

Vernon, M. and Makowsky, B. Deafness and minority group dynamics. Deaf Am, 21:3-6, 1969.

Williams, B.R. Challenge and opportunity. J Rehabil Deaf, 1:3-9, 1967.

Chapter 12

THE AMPUTEE

Case One—Triple Amputee
Case Two—Congenital Leg Amputee
Case Three—Leg Amputee
Case Four—Right Hemipelvectomy
Discussion Questions
Suggested Reading

CASE ONE – TRIPLE AMPUTEE

JOE is a 21-year-old, black, male triple amputee. He was disabled at age 13 when he was run over by a train which resulted in the loss of both his legs and his right arm. He walks with the aid of prosthetic legs and crutches.

Joe was a State Crippled Children's Clinic client from age 13 until age 21 where he received a great deal of therapy and many prosthetic devices. Vocational rehabilitation entered the picture in 1969 when he completed high school and expressed a desire for training.

As the idea of training for Joe was explored, many factors had to be taken into consideration. He was from a culturally deprived family which consisted of his mother and three younger siblings. His family existed on aid received from the welfare department and from food stamps. Testing showed him to have a verbal IQ of 87 and the culture fair IQ test yielded an IQ of 101. Due to these factors, coupled with his severe disabilities, it was determined that Joe should be placed in a comprehensive evaluation center.

In September, 1969, Joe began a two-months evaluation program at a comprehensive evaluation center. Joe adjusted quite well to the center, was extremely cooperative, showed a willingness to do anything that would help him. During the evaluation it was noted that Joe had an interest in drawing and it was the consensus of the evaluation team at the end of the evaluation that Joe should pursue a drafting course.

While Joe was in evaluation, he became involved with a girl two years his senior; she became pregnant and they married shortly before the birth of their child. This turn of events seemed to give Joe added incentive to prepare himself for earning a livelihood for himself and now for his wife and child.

In January 1970, Joe was enrolled in a private school of drafting for an 8-month training program. He completed the course in August 1970 and then he, his counselor and former instructors began looking for employment for him.

In January 1971, Joe got a temporary job as a phone solicitor which he kept until May 1971 when he got a job as a draftsman with the telephone company where he earned a salary of $60.00 per week. He kept this job for three to four weeks and then was laid off the company due to lack of work.

Joe and his counselor again began looking for employment for him as he desperately needed money to support himself and his family. During this time, Joe and his wife and child were living in the home with his mother who still had no income other than a welfare check and food stamps.

After searching diligently for months for a job for Joe, he and his counselor eventually decided that no progress was being made in securing a job for him so Joe was placed in work adjustment training at a sheltered workshop with the hope that he might eventually be placed on the payroll at that facility. Joe adjusted well to the facility and again was quite cooperative and did everything that was suggested in hope that it might be of benefit to him. Even though it was hoped that he might be hired at the sheltered workshop, the counselor continued to try to secure outside employment for Joe. At one point, Joe's counselor talked with the representative of a private employment agency and asked for his help in securing employment for Joe. The employment agency representative did find Joe a drafting job with a local contracting firm and Joe gladly accepted this position. Joe was quite pleased to get the job and immediately seemed to settle down and some of his anxiety seemed to leave and he seemed to develop a confidence that he had not shown in the past.

Joe has now been employed for approximately 12 months and receives a monthly salary of $350.00. He is pleased with his job and his employer is pleased with his work so it is felt that this will be a permanent placement. Joe and his wife, and their children which number two at this point, have bought a home and they seem to be enjoying a standard of living never known to them before.

The story of Joe was presented because it is the story of a boy who succeeded in life in spite of seemingly insurmountable obstacles. In spite of being a triple amputee, being culturally deprived and having only average intelligence, Joe coupled his tremendous motivation with the resources made available to him and has become a productive citizen.

CASE TWO – CONGENITAL LEG AMPUTEE

Memo to: D.V.R. Counselor
From: Workshop Counselor
Date: June 23, 1971
Re: Joe Smith

Joe is a good candidate for vocational rehabilitation. He is a 49-year-old with congenitally absent legs. He has a sixth grade education. He is independent in ADL and has a high potential for competitive employment. He successfully helped run a lawnmower shop for five years in Watts until it was closed after the riots.

He has his own transportation and his workshop evaluation reports excellent work habits and aptitudes.

Please see enclosed summary from his referring counselor. Advise of your action.

Thanks,

signed Workshop Counselor

SMITH, JOE

Summary

The potential for the client's self-support is excellent. His dexterity is good and so is his initiative and motivation. Mr. Smith started ETS training at the Cerebral Palsy Foundation, Whittier area, on 9/28/69. The client appeared interested in each type of assignment and spent extra time completing a task. He comprehends instructions, follows supervision quite well and was able to maintain a good relationship with fellow workers.

Mr. Smith received a 6th grade education in Sioux City, Iowa. He has always regretted not continuing with his schooling. He was at Epi-Hab, Los Angeles for six months in 1965. Later he was a trainee at Rancho Los Amigos Workshop where he remained for about 6 months. Rancho referred him to a school in Los Angeles for welding and he stayed there for 3-4 months. From 1956 to 1963 he was employed as a lawnmower repairman.

The client is a very motivated individual whose main goal is to become self-supporting and independent to our agency. Mr. Smith has an ulcer condition for which he is receiving treatment. The major diagnosis per the DA3 on file is congenital malformation of legs and right hand. Despite his physical condition, Mr. Smith drives an automobile, and uses a wheelchair and skateboard for ambulation.

Other Agency referring Counselor

Joe's application listed his disability as "No Legs." His work history showed only one job lasting 6 years as lawnmower sharpening and repair. He was being evaluated by a workshop at the time of referral. The workshop evaluation report indicated employability in following instructions, learning and retention, Productivity-Quality, adaptability with potential employable in Quantity of production. In Physical Abilities, he was rated employable in gross dexterity, sitting-prolonged, visual activity with eye-hand coordination and fine dexterity potentially employable. Work Habits were all rated employable. The case development can be followed in counselors dictated memos:

Initial Interview

Joe is a 49-year-old double amputee as a result of a congenital anomaly. He was referred to the workshop by Los Angeles Assistance Program for evaluation. He was then referred to our office by the workshop counselor and is interested in obtaining training and placement as an automotive electrician. He has done some work related to this on his own automobile, has operated a machine shop for lawnmowers for about seven years and has worked on wiring for submarines. He subsists on $114.00 a month Social Security, and $34.00 a month public assistance. He has a sixth-grade education, but feels that he doesn't have any problems reading. He knows that he can handle automotive manuals which he does. Mr. Smith rated a very good preliminary report from the workshop, has done extremely well in evaluation and is clever using his hands and brain. He was given an application to fill out and return and the workshop will send over more evaluation material. Mr. Smith seems to be a good prospect for rehabilitation.

Counselor

Case Memo, Joe Smith 8/2/70

Joe has been in the TowAway Automotive Repair School in Paramount for 10 days and appears to be progressing adequately. We should make an authorization for his tuition.

Counselor

Statement of Eligibility, Joe Smith 8/12/70

Due to the absence of both legs, Mr. Smith cannot be reasonably expected to enter competitive labor market without significant services from us. There is an excellent chance that training will render him competitively employable.

Counselor

Case Evaluation, Joe Smith 8/12/70

Joe has been evaluated at the Workshop and by the TowAway Automotive Repair School and from all accounts is a reliable, motivated candidate for services. His handicap is not too severe but that training should render him competitively employable.

Counselor

PLAN MEMORANDUM (Rehabilitation Plan)

NAME Smith, Joe   Plan to begin 8/12/70
Vocational Objective   Automatic Transmission Repairman
Approximate Date Client will Be Ready
for Employment   Febuary 1971

RATIONALE – MEDICAL – PHYSCHOLOGICAL

Proposed objective is suitable physically because lifting is not involved. Proposed objective fits very well into the client's educational and skill areas.

VOCATIONAL – EDUCATIONAL

This client has a very minimal education but has learned to read technical material on his own and should be able to be employable at the conclusion of the course.

SOCIAL – ECONOMIC

Client subsists on Social Security Disability benefits. He is single and has no outstanding debts.

DVR SERVICES

Tuition, tools and supplies – TowAway Automotive Training School
Transportation
Placement
Auto Insurance

OTHER

None

RESULTS

Client should be competitively employed at the end of training in automatic transmission repair. He has already demonstrated competency in mechanical areas in the past because he had some experience as a lawnmower repairman.

RECONCILIATION OF INFORMATION

There are no contraindications to this plan except for possible employer resistance to hiring a double-amputee for automatic transmission repair, however, this work has been successfully done by paraplegics in the past and Mr. Smith appears to be strongly motivated for employment.

Counselor

Case Memo, Joe Smith 9/15/70

Checked with teacher at the TowAway Automotive Training School Today and find that Joe is doing very well in transmission repair and that all efforts will be made at the completion of the course to place him.

Counselor

Case Memo, Joe Smith 10/14/70

Joe called in regard to his tools, he still hasn't received them, therefore, I asked him to call again Friday and if he has not received them by then, we will cancel the whole order with First Hardware and try to place the order through the school. Joe feels that he is doing okay in the course and is having no particular problems except with his automobile and he is looking around to buy another one. I have told him that we would try to help him with expenses.

Counselor

Case Memo Joe Smith 1/12/71

Effective this date this case is transferred to another counselor due to transfer of original counselor.

Counselor

Case Memo, Joe Smith 6/27/71

Since I picked up Mr. Smith's case on January 12th I have had numerous contacts with him. I have had Mr. Smith in my office for four or five lengthy visits and also have had quite a few telephone conversations with him.

When I picked up Mr. Smith's case he was not attending school at the TowAway Automotive Training School even though he had been going there previously. Mr. Smith was having some car problems and also his father had died recently. My initial work with Mr. Smith was trying to find out some type of suitable transportation for him to get back and forth to school and also to try to find out just how motivated he was to continue in his training program. Pursuant to this, I went down to the TowAway Automotive Training School to talk with the head of the school, to see just how Joe was making out in his program. In talking to the manager and looking over the school I got the impression that the school had not made a firm commitment to the former counselor about placement after Joe finished with his training program. My supervisor, who also made this visit to the training school was somewhat disturbed by the seeming lack of placement that the school had had in the past.

Mr. Smith was able to secure an automobile within approximately two months after I picked up his case. He was able to outfit this car so that he could drive it without the use of his legs. It was a joint decision of both Joe and myself that he could not really learn anything more down at the TowAway Automotive Training School and therefore there was no reason for him to continue going there.

Following this, my supervisor and I had Mr. Smith in my office for a discussion to see just what he could do with his training and how much he knew about automobile transmission work. Joe seemed to have all the skills necessary to be an automobile transmission expert and the problem seems to be to find a place for him to work. It was decided after this conference that he would try to use what resources he could, in the Paramount area to see if he could find someone who would take him on an OJT program or straight work assignment. My supervisor and I both decided that a good approach would be to try to contact one of the big employers to see if they would have a place where they could absorb Joe in their plants. On trying to contact a couple of the large manufacturers here it was found that there was no way for Joe to gain an entry-level job. I personally have contacted Ace Motor Company here in Los Angeles and also Arco Distributors to see if there was anything that Joe could do and the response has been negative.

Joe hasn't seemed to be able to followup on his end of the contract in that he does not seem to have made any contact with any of the local employers. Joe claims that he has spent every day for the last two months looking for employment but that employers always reject him because of his physical disabilities. However, when I try to find out what places he has been to, he does not have any names or organizations that he can speak of. During this past month it has been impossible to contact Joe at home since he is out everyday. He says that he has been looking for a job but as I mentioned above he never indicates what places or individuals he has spoken to. I have begun to have strong feelings that Joe is having some problem with alcoholism since on quite a few visits into my office he has smelled of alcohol and also he cannot account for his whereabouts during the day. However, upon confronting Joe with this he denies that he has any problem in drinking and that he only has an occasional beer. I am really not quite certain in my own mind whether Joe is telling the truth or not. Therefore, I have told Joe that from now on when he checks with any employers he should get the names of individuals that he has spoken to. I have asked him to do this so that I can check back and see if Joe is spending his time looking for employment or whether he is just out drinking and not really being honest about where he has been spending his time. At this point, I am pretty much in a quandary as to just what to do with him. The problem with Mr. Smith is that he might be able to do transmission work but there does not seem to be anyone at this time who is willing to take a chance on him or as mentioned above he might have such a problem with alcohol that he couldn't be a steady employee.

Even if Joe does not have a problem with alcohol, it has been indicated in some of his past jobs that he has quit out of sheer frustration with his employer and has a very low burning point. At first, I thought it might be a good idea to try to evaluate Joe here in the workshop but he has been evaluated here and in fact has been trained by our office in Paramount in welding and he stayed at a school in Los Angeles for three to four months and quit for some reason that only he knows. Also from 1956 to 1963 he was employed as a lawnmower repairmen.

At this point I am trying to put together all of the previous jobs Joe has held and also the previous training that the Department has helped him with to see if we cannot come up with some type of a job for him. I have spent quite a lot of time with Mr. Smith trying to figure out just what type of a vocational goal would be best for him and we do not seem to be getting anywhere. In my last conversation with Mr. Smith, I told him that I would probably be closing his case within a couple of months if we could not find some type of suitable employment since we did not seem to be making any progress. He was amenable to this suggestion and said that he hoped that we could find something within the next two months. Since I made that statement to Mr. Smith he seems to be trying to come up with some ideas as to what he can do.

Counselor

Case Memo, Joe Smith 7/7/71

Since my last dictation with Mr. Smith's case, I have had a couple of conversations with him and have decided that the best way to evaluate Mr. Smith's skills might be at All Careers School with a three week brush-up course, which is given by Mr. Mature. Mr. Mature has met with Joe during the past week and feels that there is a feasible chance that with a three-week brush-up course he could place him, therefore, I am going to authorize $79.00 per week for three weeks for Mr. Smith at All Careers School for training in small appliance repair.

An additional purpose of this brush-up is to determine if the client will get to school on time. He will have time to apply for jobs on leads furnished by the school. His attendance will help determine whether his personal habits will interfere with his ability to work.

Counselor

PLAN MEMORANDUM (Plan Addenda)

NAME <u>SMITH, Joe</u>　　　　　　Plan to Begin <u>7/10/71</u>
Vocational Objective <u>Small appliance repair</u>
Approximate Date Client Will Be Ready
　　　　　　　for Employment <u>7/31/71</u>

Effective 7/10/71, I am authorizing $79.00 per week for three weeks to Mr. Mature at All Careers School for Joe Smith, Mr. Mature has agreed that if he is not able to place Mr. Smith at the end of three weeks of training he will not charge the department anything. This training will be for small appliance repair.

For rationale see Case memo dated 7/7/71.

Counselor

Case Memo Joe Smith 8/21/71

As indicated in my dictation of July 7, 1971 I started Joe in All Career School for a brush-up course in small appliance repair. Joe did very well in his attendance and work there.

After Joe's training, with the help of Mr. Mature, I was able to find a place where he could use his skills that he had learned not only at the All Careers School but also at the TowAway Automotive Training School. He began working on the 14th of August at Paramount Mower & Saw Company, 11410 Brooks, Paramount, California. The owner is Mr. Peter Cook.

During a meeting I had with Mr. Smith in my office on the 21st of August he indicated that things were going along fairly well at his new job and he did not foresee any problems as of this date. Joe told me that he was working on different types of motors and also working on sharpening some lawnmowers. He told me that he was making $2.50 an hour for a forty-hour week. He said that he usually worked Tuesdays through Saturdays and can sometime get work on Monday and usually averages anywhere from $100.00 to $120.00 a week depending upon how many hours he works. Because of the problem that Joe has with his lung we have talked to his boss, Mr. Cook, and asked him to keep Joe away from doing too much work in the sharpening department, which would only aggravate his physical condition. This company does a lot of work for the city of Paramount and also does some work on private vehicles.

I plan on going down to the company within the next two weeks to talk to Joe about how it is going on the job and also talk to Mr. Cook about the possibility of hiring some other individuals in his shop. Joe told me that he has no trouble getting around in the shop and uses his skateboard to get in and out and when he is doing his work, he uses a high stool that they have fixed up for him. The job that Joe is now in seems to be something that he can handle and if after visiting the shop in a couple of weeks I do not see any problems in Joe being permanently employed there I will probably be closing his case as rehabilitated.

Counselor

Case Memo, Joe Smith 9/1/71

Contact with Paramount Mower and Saw Company this morning indicates that Joe is still working there and doing well.

The Amputee

After reviewing Mr. Smith's case I decided it might be important to give some of the rationale behind why I decided not to fit him with prosthetic devices and also why I decided not to encourage him to give up his use of the skateboard for a wheelchair. In looking through Mr. Smith's case and also in the numerous contacts I had with Mr. Smith before my dictation of the 27th of June I came to realize that this man had a life style that had been built up over 50 years of living with his disability. Mr. Smith has been congenitally disabled since birth. Both of his legs were amputated at a very early age in the small town that Joe grew up in and they did not have very extensive medical facilities, therefore, during Joe's early childhood he was never considered a candidate for any type of prosthetic devices.

I discussed with Joe, on a couple of occasions, the possibility that prosthetic devices might make it more functionally able for him to work and also might make his appearance more cosmetically pleasing. However, he indicated to me that since the stumps of his legs were so short, only approximately three inches long, and also since he had lived almost his entire life by getting around on different types of skateboards that he did not want to mess around with legs at this late age.

In considering Mr. Smith's whole life history and life style up until I picked his case, I decided that it would be best not to pressure anything on this man since he was 50 years of age and did not seem too concerned about his appearance but was more concerned in trying to find a job that he could handle. Also, I think it should be indicated that I discussed with Joe the possibility of him using a wheelchair and found that he has one but that he did not like to use it because it got in his way when he was working around motors and also he had a lot more difficulty in transporting it back and forth in his automobile. After observing Joe in my office in his wheelchair and also on his skateboard and also observing him on different training sites using both of these devices I would agree that the skateboard for this man makes a lot more sense even though it might not look as cosmetically pleasing to some individuals.

Another thing to take into consideration in Mr. Smith's case is the fact that time is important to him and therefore it was very important to find a job that he could do that would give him immediate gratification in the form of money and that would not involve an extensive training program. This is based upon the fact that Joe has been used to fending for himself since an early age and does not have much tolerance for long range goals.

It takes Joe about 3 to 5 minutes to unload his wheelchair and get in it when he is using it while it takes him from 1 to 3 minutes to use his skateboard. Also, he can get around on his skateboard in much smaller areas and this is important not only in the work that he is now doing but was important in his training and is also important at his home in that he is able to work on his own automobile, he is able to get around in his own kitchen and take care of his own needs where a wheelchair, because of the space it takes up, would create more of a problem. What I more or less did with Mr. Smith was give him the alternative and let him choose for himself and I think that he made the best decision.

Also in trying to place this individual I realized right from the beginning that he was not an individual who would be overly concerned with his appearance and therefore could probably not perform clerical duties as I first thought might be good for him. To clarify that a little bit, it should be said that Mr. Smith could physically perform clerical duties but does not have either the patience or the social persuasiveness to work at a desk eight hours a day. Mr. Smith does not have much of a frustration tolerance in working with people but does appear to have a good tolerance in working with things, particularly things that he can build, such as motors and other types of electronic and mechanical devices. Two of the reasons that I focused intensely on placement with Mr. Smith were, first of all his age, which does not give him that much longer workable years and therefore it would be foolish to put him through an extensive training program. I think the second, and most important is the fact that Mr. Smith is a man who has a lot of pride in being able to make his own living and therefore probably would not benefit much from intensified counseling but would benefit a lot from someone who would help him to design the type of equipment that he would need to function at his job. One also has to observe Mr. Smith in his everyday activities to see how he is able to perform with the use of his skateboard and the

The Amputee

high stool that he now uses at work. Basically, Joe uses an approach that probably is all wrong from a so-called pure way of manipulating the use of his body to bring about maximum functional ability. However, Mr. Smith's way works for him and therefore I think it would be quite silly to try to ask him to use a procedure that might look good but wouldn't aid in his vocational development or help him with his activities of daily living. I think that this is a case where if something works for the individual, the counselor should not interfere since he might create a lot of problems that the client never had before.

This memo will give some idea of the rationale behind what I did with Mr. Smith and why I think that he is still successfully employed to this day and should be able to maintain the job he holds now unless there is some erotic change in his behavior.

Counselor

Evaluation

This case study was chosen as it illustrates the value of a common sense evaluation of a disabled person's life style. The counselor did not try to impose on the client his own need for the client to wear prosthesis. With 3-inch stumps and at his age any attempt to fit him with prosthesis would probably have ended in failure. The mobility of the client on his skateboard is fast and efficient, in fact, he moves around faster than most persons walk.

The case also illustrates the fact that there may be many vocational acitvities a disabled person can satisfactorily perform but employers may not be willing to give the disabled a chance to perform them. The transmission repair objective may have been quite feasible as far as the physical demands go but the placement aspects had not been carefully evaluated.

The reader will note the client was placed in about the same kind of work he had performed before. Vocational history tends to repeat itself.

CASE THREE – LEG AMPUTEE

John Reso applied for rehabilitation service in 1964. He was 52 years old and had worn an AK prosthesis since age of 28. He was injured in a cavein which resulted in comminuted fractures of all the bones of his leg. He has a 4-inch stump remaining. Mr. Reso lived with his wife and was forced to seek public assistance during this period of unemployment. His educational level was eighth grade; however, his work history revealed that he had considerable skill as a precision grinder (even though he could not spell "precision" he was able to earn up to $6.50 per hour). The client was not tested nor was there any attempt to improve his formal education.

He requested the agency to purchase a new prosthesis for him as his present prosthesis was cracked and deteriorated to the point that no suitable repairs could be made. He also wanted placement help. His present prosthesis was purchased by a rehabilitation agency in an eastern state. (As his original injury was an industrial accident it is assumed that a lump sum settlement was made as a replacement of prosthesis is normally a part of any negotiated industrial accident settlement.)

John was usually employed as a machine operator, a job that required him to be on his feet most of the day, walking or standing. He was sent to an orthopedist for a prescription. The physician reported,

> his present leg is three-and-a-half years old, a total contact suction socket with a pull-on sock. The socket is wooden with a free knee and has never had any type friction or lock knee. He uses a hip control belt.

The gait was generally acceptable with a slight left lurch and John likes to have the knee snapped back into full hyperextension. Inspection of the stump revealed a four-inch stump with a well-healed scar and an area of maceration over the erolateral ischial seat on the left. The range of motion of left hip extension was 10°, flexion 100°, abduction 30°, adduction 20°. There were no tender superficial sites. The prescription,

> left AK prosthesis with quadrilateral suction socket, free nonfriction, nonlocking knee. Conventional ankle (as present) and either conventional or Sach foot. Hip control belt.

A financial survey revealed that John was unemployed at the time of his application but had obtained a job prior to authorization for the prosthesis. During his period of unemployment he had gone into debt, which was considered in determining his financial eligibility. The new prosthesis was ordered from firm number one. Firm number one had made John's old prosthesis.

Medical information obtained showed our client was a diabetic since 1942 and took 30 units of Lente 40 insulin a day. The patient thinks he is well controlled but inquiry by the vocational counselor revealed that he had not consulted his doctor for three-and-one-half years. He also had glaucoma. The client was urged to stay with medical supervision. A dental examination revealed extensive pyorrhea with a recommendation of full upper extraction and a complete denture. In a note to the district medical consultant the counselor wrote:

A. Absence of left leg AK   # 898
   Pyorrhea   # 532.1
   Diabetes Mellitus   # 260
   Glaucoma   # 387

B. The absent left leg limits the client's mobility and physical capabilities (including lifting) which are essential for normal work and daily living activities. The pyorrhea, diabetes and glaucoma are not disabling at the present time, but could be if appropriate medical care is not obtained.

C. It is recommended that an appropriate prosthesis be purchased by our department. The recommended dental work can also be financed by D.R. Since the diabetes and glaucoma are continuous medical problems which could be disabling, the client should be urged to personally obtain adequate and continuous medical supervision. The new prosthesis will immediately increase the client's function in daily living and work activities. The dental work should alleviate any further dental problems. Continuous medical supervision can reduce potential disabilities which might result from the diabetes and glaucoma.

— signed counselor —

The Medical Consultant wrote:

To assure he remains under medical supervision I recommend that we get progress reports re: glaucoma and diabetes at three month's intervals from his physician. First report should be requested now"

Medical Consultant

Company number one ran into difficulties in fitting Mr. Reso. Three sockets were made. The client after receiving the last one wrote the orthopedist.

Dear Dr.

I am writting you this letter in regard to the prosthesis I am wearing.

1. The valve is not working properly, it leaks.

2. It is too high. I cannot reach the floor with my hands stretched down.

3. It pinches me.

4. I am not getting proper suction.

Doctor, this prosthesis is not made properly. It should be made over. I will explain this to you next week.

Yours truly,

J. Reso

The doctor's recheck found the fit unsatisfactory reporting "inadequate flexion built into the socket with anterior brim too high."

Company number one, by this time, had run out of patience saying the problem was a short stump. They reported having built three other prosthesis for this man and he complained about all of them. Company number one told Mr. Reso to return the prosthesis and they would cancel the department's purchase authorization. The orthopedist on a second recheck indicated the prosthesis was not satisfactory due to "adduction roll and excess ischial pressure." The orthopedist suggested that another prosthetist try to fit the client.

The client went to company number two who evaluated the ill-fitting prosthesis. They reported:

Suction: Adequate
Abduction: Angle too severe

Posterior Seat: Slopes medially allowing patient to slide onto public ramus
Anterior Brim: Too low allowing roll to hang out
Pelvic Belt: Should be changed along with socket
General Alignment of Prosthesis: Satisfactory. Recommend new quad socket and pelvic band with hip joint aligned to present prosthesis

Company number one took back the prosthesis and cancelled the authorization. Another purchase authorization was sent to company number two. The second prosthesis was a satisfactory fit. John arranged for medical supervision of his glaucoma and diabetes after his counselor pointed out some dire future developments that could occur. John Reso's final prosthesis was an excellent fit. He obtained a job as machinest and was very happy with his prosthesis. Case was closed "rehabilitated."

Evaluation

This case study was chosen because of the counselor's demonstration of his understanding of the medical factors. It is also interesting to note that he wrote in paragraph C (to the Medical Consultant) "the new prosthesis will immediately increase the client's function in daily living and work activities." The order is quite proper and many times counselors become so work-oriented that they overlook the daily living problems.

The case also indicates that there is much of the "Art" left in the prosthetist's work as well as scientific know how. Prosthetists may vary in their ability to fit certain kinds of cases and the counselor shouldn't become upset when he runs into such a problem. The main problem, as it is in most amputee cases, was in the proper fit of the prosthesis.

Evidently there was no amputee conference team available in the area that could have assisted the original prosthetist in solving the fitting problems. The delay caused by the fitting problem may have been avoided if the two companies had been willing to work together on fitting problems.

CASE FOUR – RIGHT HEMIPELVECTOMY

Creed Botei, an experienced auto mechanic of 20 years, noticed a swelling on his upper right thigh. When the condition persisted he went to a doctor. He was then referred to a hospital for a biopsy. At this time Mr. Boter was working, earning $1000 a month. Lacking sufficient funds to pay for the extensive surgery, he was referred to a private charitable hospital for treatment and rehabilitation services.

The biopsy proved to be malignant and a right hemipelvectomy was performed. Mr. Boter was 35 years of age, a single Caucasian, who had worked in foreign countries as an auto mechanic before migrating to the United States. He was single but had many friends in his home area. He applied for Social Security and his benefit amounted to $194.00 a month which provided for basic living needs. His educational level was ninth grade but he had no language problems. His work history and earnings record revealed that he was a skilled mechanic who was able to maintain steady employment until the problem arose with his leg.

The counselor's recording is as follows:

Case Memorandum, Creed Boter, 9/2/70

This is a 35-year-old, rather obese, Caucasian male who was referred to us through HRD prior to the Social Security referral. He currently receives state disability benefits but has applied for SSDI. The form D831 indicates that he has been certified as under a disability since May 1, 1970.

Education After elementary school in Austria, his native country, he attended three years of trade school to become an auto mechanic. He has remained in that occupation until the time of his surgery.

Work History His only employment has been in auto mechanics, and his employment record shows a good work record in that field from Austria, Canada and United States. At the time of his surgery he states he was making $1,000 per month working for a local garage that specializes in foreign car repair.

Presenting Disability In June 1970, this individual underwent a right hemipelvectomy for liposarcoma. Medical records from Charity Hospital indicate that they are attempting to fit him with a prosthesis, but in counselor's opinion, at this level a prosthesis will be more a hindrance than a help. If he is ever going to be able to work in anything related to the automotive field, I envision some sort of a high seat walker, especially constructed to accommodate him in an almost erect position. Possibly because it is so soon after surgery it appears that he has some difficulty sitting in any one position for any length of time now. For this reason it would seem that a sedentary occupation might not be appropriate.

General Impression and Expectations and Abilities of Client This is a very strongly motivated individual who has always worked at his trade and he is determined to become self-supporting once again. At present, he ambulates with crutches and it is my feeling that this will be more effective than any prosthesis could ever be at this level. I would like to have field time to visit his most recent employer and evaluate whether or not a special walker could be made for Mr. Boter, by the means of which he would be able to continue in some phases of his former occupation. Our State Technical Consultant will be consulted in this regard if it seems at all possible that he can do some of the operations of the job.

Case Memorandum, 2/14/71

Case Evaluation and Eligibility Statement

This is a 35-year-old single, Caucasian male who has had a right hip disarticulation as a result of cancer. He is being seen in followup at the Charity Hospital where a prosthesis was provided. His physician has indicated it would be appropriate for client to return to employment after February 29, 1971, and recommends that he use a motorized wheelchair. This client has had twenty years experience in auto mechanics, and his former employer will be willing to hire him if he has an electric wheelchair instead of walking with the prosthesis and crutches on the cement shop floor, which may have oil spots anywhere and everywhere. I have spoken to both the former employer and the doctor in order to ascertain medical approval, as well as employer acceptance, of his return to employment.

This individual does have a medically diagnosed disability, namely, amputation of right extremity at hip which is a handicap to his employment as an auto mechanic which he has done continually for the past twenty years. There is a reasonable expectation that the services of this agency (provision of electric wheelchair) will render this individual fit to engage in a gainful occupation because: a) work is part of his life style and he is very strongly motivated to return to employment, b) his former employer regards his work very highly and is willing to accept him as a supervisor in a sedentary capacity providing the individual has an electric wheelchair, c) his doctor sent us a written recommendation and approval for Mr. Boter to return to work after February 29.

2-25-71

Even though Mr. Boter has been provided a prosthesis at Charity Hospital, understandably he finds it much too cumbersome and prefers to use crutches with which he ambulated much more freely. Therapists there did recommend he use a wheelchair, and his former employer is willing to rehire him as a supervisor of auto mechanics at the foreign car dealership here in Los Angeles if he does have an electric wheelchair. It is obvious that either the prosthesis or crutches would be very hazardous on the shop floor. Mr. Boter has been to several dealers to evaluate the type of chair that will be most suitable for him and for his occupation. I have conferred with our technical consultant if it should prove a necessity on the job.

A plan will be written to provide this client with the electric wheelchair which will enable him to become employed and once again self-supporting.

PLAN MEMORANDUM

Rehabilitation Plan   Extended Evaluation Plan   Plan Addenda
NAME BOTER, Creed   Plan to Begin At Once
Vocational Objective   Auto Mechanic Supervisor
Approximate Date Client Will be Ready
                for Employment   March 10, 1972

Justification

See Memo   2/25/71

DR Services to be Provided

Electric wheelchair as recommended by doctor at Charity Hospital and required by prospective employer.

Services Provided by Other Agencies

SSDI – $194.40 per month.

Charity Hospital
> Crutch Walking
> Gait Training
> Loan of Walker
> How to Fall
> Home Checkout
> Out-Patient Follow-up Care

Rehabilitation Counselor   2-25-71   Rehabilitation Supervisor

After consultation with the Medical Consultant regarding his recommendations the counselor agreed that continuing supervision of Charity Hospital was needed. Our Medical Consultant approved of the purchase of a motorized wheelchair. The discharge summary and the excellent after-care on which he made his decision are reproduced:

DISCHARGE SUMMARY

PATIENT   Boter, Creed   HOSPITAL   42-31-04
ADMITTED   6-4-70   DISCHARGED   6-24-70

Final Diagnosis LIPOSARCOMA RIGHT THIGH

Operation RIGHT PELVECTOMY (Hemi)

History This is the first Charity Hospital admission of a 35-year-old Caucasian male, who was worked up as an out-patient with the history of liposarcoma of right thigh. The patient was tentatively scheduled for a hemipelvectomy and IVP showed a possible deviation of the ureter on the right and this is being evaluated prior to consideration of the right hemipelvectomy. This patient has a known mass in the right thigh for one month and was biopsied two weeks previously showing the liposarcoma.

Physical Examination Well-developed, obese, Caucasian male in no acute distress. Blood pressure 132/80. Head — normocephalic Lungs clear to P. & A. Heart — regular sinus rhythm, no murmurs. Abdomen — soft, obese, no masses or tenderness. There is some indication of small nodes in the right groin. Extremities — there is a large 20 X 30 xm. mass in the posterior medial aspect of the right thigh. Rectal negative.

Laboratory Data 1 — 3 WBC's in the urine per high-power field, white blood count 6,900, hemoglobin 12.3, hematocrit 37.5 with 69

segs, 14 lymphs, 7 monos, 6 eosinophils.

Hospital Course The patient was taken to surgery on 6-9-70, where an excision was made in the right groin to evaluate the right ureter. There was no deviation of the ureter and no cause for deviation. The wound was closed and operation was continued on as a right hemipelvectomy. The nodes on rapid frozen section were benign for any metastatic process. Post operatively the patient did well. The suction catheters were removed on the third post operative day. The patient complained of pain in the area and some phantom pains were at times painful to the patient. Phantom pain was controlled with percodan. The patient was instructed by physical therapy regarding crutch walking and was also shown how to fall. The patient was discharged on the fourteenth post operative day apparently able to handle things quite well and was ambulating well in the ward with the use of crutches. Home Health will make follow-up visits to his home to evaluate this patient and he will return to see us in the clinic in one week to be continued for evaluation and followed as an out-patient.

Resident Surgeon
6/29/70

Home Health Service

Boter, Creed

H.V. Home evaluation visit made as requested. No evidence of patient at home. Front and back doors locked, front screen door unlatched. No response to phone call.

Later checked with Social Service and nursing personnel, all of whom believe his plan was to go to his home. Also, all stated he had many friends who visited regularly, and that he probably was staying with one of them.

Registered Nurse
6-25-70

Home Health Service

Boter, Creed

H.V. Patient home alone. Says he is managing "pretty good". Looked tired. Said he had tried to mow the lawn with power mower, but mower kept getting away from him. Would like a walker for a week or two until he is able to get to the shop and weld the walker he plans making for himself. Says a friend will install supports in bathroom so he can get in and out of tub shower. Suggested he get tub seat. Also advised removal of small loose rug in bathroom. Will arrange for walker through A.C.S.

Registered Nurse
6-28-70

Home Health Service

Boter, Creed
Visited patient at home to discuss resources available for recreational swimming. Reviewed sleeping pattern and habits. Suggestions were given to aid patient to re-establish nighttime sleeping.

Occupational Therapist
7-16-70

The prescription below permitted the client to return to work and approved the use of an electric powered wheelchair.

Dear Counselor,

In reply to your question regarding Mr. Boter's ability to return to work, I believe it would be advisable for him to do so at any time after February 29, 1971, especially if he has the use of a motorized wheelchair.

Sincerely,

CHARITY HOSPITAL RESIDENT

Case Memorandum, Boter, Creed   4/24/71

Mr. Boter today called to tell me about his wheelchair breaking down and having to be returned for repairs. The vendor has given him a loaner which is not operating properly, either due to a malfunctioning battery or some electrical deficiency. He said he had tried to get from the manufacturer a copy of the schematics on this particular wheelchair because he felt that he himself would be able to make future repairs. I told him that our first step should be to immediately call the vendor to explain to them about this loaner wheelchair being inadequate and the next step would be for me to check with our technical consultant to find out whether or not this schematic for the electrical system for this wheelchair could be obtained from any other source. I did call the vendor and told him very firmly that we were paying for the almost $1,000 chair, which is now in for repair and I felt it was only proper that Mr. Boter be furnished an adequate powered wheelchair during the time the newly purchased one is in for repairs. I was assured that they would take care of this today.

I did telephone the technical consultant to ask if he had any leads as to how the schematics for the electrical system on this battery powered wheelchair could be secured. He told me that he knows of no way one could obtain same. He stated that this is a very closely guarded secret, since it cost the manufacturer many thousands of dollars to develop this particular system, and they are very jealously guarding their secret.

Case Memorandum, Boter, Creed   4/26/71

Checked with vendor again to be sure of loaner. He has another. The manufacturer is replacing a module in the chair we are purchasing.

Case Memorandum (Closure Memorandum)   5/26/71

The client's wheelchair was delivered to his place of employment on 4/3/71, and Mr. Boter was immediately on the job, part-time initially. I have spoken to his employer, Mr. Jones, and he is very delighted to have Mr. Boter back on the job. We discussed whether or not it would be necessary to have a special lower bench prepared for Mr. Boter to use for work, but Mr. Jones tells me that the facilities they have right now are perfectly adequate. Much of Mr. Boter's work is done at the bench, but with his electric wheelchair, he is able to get about the shop to advise other mechanics and confer on mechanical problems anywhere in the shop. Since this client has been enabled to return to his former employment by this agency's having provided him with the essential electric wheelchair required for mobility on the job, I feel justified in closing this case in status 26. Mr. Boter now earns $200 a week.

This case was chosen because it illustrated in a very fine way the coordination often needed to complete a rehabilitation. Charity

Hospital had no funds for the powered wheelchair. The followup home visits are so essential to determine the quality of function in the home. The creativeness of the counselor in thinking specifically about the work area even to the point of having a specially designed walker is quite remarkable. The counselor consulted with the medical consultant and the technical consultant who offered to design the walker if needed and any special desk or work area. The counselor realized that the effort of propelling a regular wheelchair is eventually transmitted to the posterior of the wheelchair user and this was already a problem area. She added mobility and safety lessening the energy requirements, paving the way for long-term vocational activities.

DISCUSSION QUESTIONS

1. What types of jobs should be avoided by amputees?
2. Discuss various types of mechanical assistive devices that are used by amputees.
3. Discuss the "phantom limb" phenomenon.
4. Discuss the need for gait training prior to vocational planning.

SUGGESTED READING

Abram, Harry S., (Ed.) Psychological Aspects of Surgery. Boston, Little, Brown and Company, 1967.

Anderson, Miles H., et al. Prosthetic Principles, Above-Knee Amputations. Springfield, Thomas, 1960.

Blakeslee, Berton (Ed.) The Limb Deficient Child. Berkeley, University of California Press, 1963.

Lowman, Edward and Klinger, Judith L. Aides to Independent Living, Self Help for the Handicapped. New York, McGraw-Hill Book Company, 1969.

Step into Action – A Guidebook for the Above-Knee Amputee. No. 980, U.S. Department of Health, Education, and Welfare in collaboration with Department of Surgery and Institute of Rehabilitation Medicine, New York University Medical Center, 1964.

The Geriatric Amputee, No. 919, Committee on Prosthetics Research and Development, National Academy of Sciences, National Research Council, Washington, D.C., 1961.

Tosberg, William A. Upper and Lower Extremity Prostheses. Springfield, Thomas, 1962.

Chapter 13

RHEUMATOID ARTHRITIS

Discussion Questions
Suggested Reading

DAVID Willson, as his Biblical namesake, was a small but mighty guy. As a boy he was very active in baseball, basketball, track and other sports. He had a lot of determination, which he was going to need to face the pain and effort in store for him at age 57 when rheumatoid arthritis struck hard at his knees and feet, and later, his hands. This had been coming on gradually over the last few years, and his employment in a large factory had been progressively lighter work as a mixer, machinist, sweeper and watchman. Now there were no lighter jobs available because of automation eliminating many hand processes.

Finally, one time when he got up at night, aching, he couldn't walk because the knee hurt so bad. He decided to call the doctor, who met him at the emergency room of the hospital and gave him a shot of cortisone. David was to be on duty as a guard on the midnight shift, but he called that he wouldn't be in till the next shift. There was pain in his feet, but he felt he had to walk.

He put up with this for several months until it became so troublesome that he agreed to go into the hospital for a week. He felt better by being off his feet for a week and thought he could go back to work as a sweeper. He had a shot of cortisone in both insteps.

That weekend he went fishing. He loved to go fishing even more than he loved to talk and play cards and often combined all three; but that was the time when the pain stabbed so hard that he had to be brought home. He couldn't get up or down.

He wanted to go to Mayo's, but his doctor said he would call in an arthritis specialist first. He began treatment with gold shots. A physiatrist also examined him and prescribed exercises and heat

treatments, pulleys, exercycle and walking to keep moving.
The physiatrist's report begins,

> This 58 year-old-man gives a history of arthritis for about one year. It is interesting that the rather abrupt onset of his arthritic symptoms followed the loss of his son (he was the oldest son, and they were very close), and in the past one sees onset of arthritis following severe emotional trauma. He worked until about six months ago as a watchman but has been unable to work since April. Originally the discomfort began in his right knee, and over a period gradually developed into involvement of the ankles and feet and both knees as well as his elbows, wrists and interphalangeal joints of his hand. He has been on numerous medications without too much relief but recently has been on a series of gold injections, and although he is not in remission he appears considerably improved over what he had been from a symptomatic and objective point of view. He is now able to do many of the various activities of daily living, although he has needed some help in moving about and dressing and undressing because of the severe involvement of the joints. This, however, appears to be improving. ... I certainly think that employment is a reasonable goal to shoot for and the program as outlined above should be continued in order to achieve this goal. He is presently on an active program, so the DVR involvement could conceivably be as part of in-patient and also to continue on out-patient therapy and treatment. I believe that vocational exploration any time now would be indicated in order to develop his interests and also his attitudes and aptitudes.

DVR records show the following entries by the Counselor:

Sept. 29	Following VNA referral (she only knew name) I contacted the doctor who informed me that client had rheumatoid arthritis and would probably be able to return to work after a couple of months' treatment. He gave permission to visit client in the hospital. Admission date was September 1.
Oct. 2 Status 00 Referral Status 02 Diagnostic	An application was obtained. A General Medical Report was authorized and left with the chart as per doctor's recommendation. Client did not know who the company hospital insurance was with, and I obtained permission to get this from the hospital. Client is white, lives with

his wife in a well kept home they owned for 3 years. Their 4 children are grown and married and living nearby, with 19 grandchildren and 3 great grandchildren. His last year's income was $4400 and next year's expected income is $3000. David is a high school graduate, worked for several grocery companies, and operated his own fruit store business for four years before going into the factory 20 years ago.

Oct. 3   The hospital credit office gave the name of the insurance company. Check with doctor's secretary Wednesday about his report.

Oct. 4   General Medical Report of examination done Oct. 3 by an internist was received. His diagnosis was acute rheumatoid arthritis, and he recommended physical therapy, gold shots as an in-patient and physiatrist's consultation.

Oct. 5   Paid General Medical Bill.

Oct. 9   DVR Medical Consultant recommended physiatrist's referral to answer the question, "Will the proposed treatment actually improve the patient's condition substantially?"

Oct. 17 Counselor referred the patient to a physiatrist, included a General Medical Report and asked for an early appointment.

Oct. 25 Called physiatrist regarding his report. He stated it is completed and will be forwarded soon.

Oct. 31 The physiatrist delivered his report in person stating the voucher will follow. He thinks client is a young enough man that rehabilitation will do him some good and improve him to a point where he may be able to handle a realistic job. He recommends we follow the physical therapy on an in-patient program already instituted and vocational exploration. He should be staff with state medical consultant.

Rheumatoid Arthritis

Nov. 1 — Agency medical consultant recommended 30 days' hospitalization plus out-patient followup as recommended by the internist. He explained that this type of disability is usually chronic with exacerbations, which are considered acute when they occur, and the best time to treat is during the acute phase. Put in Status 10, ready for services.

Nov. 3 — Received voucher from physiatrist.

Nov. 7
Status 10
Plan Development
Status 16
Physical Restoration

Paid physiatrist. Completed certification of acceptance as eligible for DVR services. Counselor approved rehabilitation plan for treatment and vocational exploration.

Nov. 8 — Counselor wrote client a letter notifying him of DVR acceptance for treatment services effective Nov. 7. Report of Action sent to VNA, the referral source. Called internist. He plans to let client go home the first of the week. He has made considerable improvement and can now get around fairly well, although he still has some pain. When first seen, he could hardly move. The doctor would like for DVR to talk to the employer and arrange some sort of sheltered work where he wouldn't need fine finger or hand dexterity, but only gross movement. He feels night watchman or guard would be appropriate if he didn't have *too* much walking, but he doesn't want him to sit down too much either. Doctor thinks he will be ready to go back to work in several months at present rate. Agrees with testing and possible placement with State if client cannot get back to the factory. Doctor would like a copy of physiatrist's report.

Nov. 8 — Called doctor's nurse to find out how much gold treatments will cost and if he will need any regulatory medication; she could not tell. Will call Thursday.

Nov. 9	Doctor's secretary called. Gold treatments are $3.00 each, one every two weeks. He does not need any regulatory medication now.
Dec. 1	Received report from Federal Disability Program, allowing disability benefits.
Dec. 27	Bill received from hospital. The balance after insurance payments would be taken care of by DVR authorization, dated Nov. 7 for the remaining 9 days' hospitalization, which is actually much less than the per diem cost. Bill should be cancelled and remainder sent to the hospital.
Dec. 28	Send physician's report form for hospital treatment and letter to internist regarding outcome of hospitalization: "I was just informed that Mr. Willson was discharged from the hospital on Nov. 16, and as it has been some time since we have heard anything regarding his status, I wonder if you would be so kind as to comment on the results of treatment to date, what to expect regarding return to work, functional limitations, and any recommendations you have for further treatment. The enclosed form may facilitate this."
Jan. 8	Received physician's report from internist: Continue gold treatment; possibly in two months may return to work, by March or "whenever he feels he is able." He is "poorly motivated, could perhaps do sheltered work now." Appointment letter was sent to client.
Jan. 23	Client was in for his appointment. He was observed to have considerable difficulty walking back to my office. But in view of the doctor's report that he was somewhat poorly motivated, I questioned him regarding working and his plans for the future. He informed me that he still has considerable difficulty walking and using his hands, however, he definitely would like to return to work and would like to return to the factory where he worked for 20 years. He did not seem interested in employment as a security guard at a hotel because he feels he could make more money, $2.85 an hour sweeping at the factory. He

will contact me for assistance along this line, if needed. He has been going for physical therapy sessions every Monday, Wednesday and Friday since Dec. 22, as an out-patient and has been treated by the physiatrist with ultra-sound to both knees and shoulders. (The doctor did not inform us of this so some followup will have to be done to rectify this for he seems to be getting along all right.) I observed him leaving the building to verify the fact that he would have difficulty walking. His gait was very restricted even though he did not know he was being watched, so I have no reason to doubt his creditability.

Jan. 24   Discussed possible back dating services with Doctor. Will do, but should inform doctor that we should always be contacted prior to any service. The Doctor was called but, could not be reached, so word was left with secretary regarding information on dates and types of services performed, and regulations on requiring authorization prior to service. She will have doctor call.

Jan. 26   Called doctor again. He is out of town but his office will take care of it as it was urgent.

Feb. 8   Doctor has as yet failed to call even though he has been contacted several times. Will try to straighten this out. Trust fund eligibility verification received and certified by counselor.

Feb. 9   Called doctor regarding the reported physical therapy sessions to date. He stated that he prescribed P.T. as of the date of discharge which he could not recall off-hand. From this date on, he estimated approximately 10 additional visits. He feels that if we could authorize P.T. sessions back dated, we would probably have covered everything.

Mar. 3   Received bill from internist. Called doctor, and nurse states insurance paid $29.40 of total hospital bill of $310.00. Client will need additional treatment.

Mar. 7	Called internist's office for clarification of billing. Nurse states bill submitted as he has used up the authorization, but client will need more; and usual course runs about 20 treatments. He hasn't submitted office visits because insurance usually doesn't take care of this. I informed her that the insurance forms should be presented prior to our paying, so I shall return the bill for action. She will check with the doctor to see how many additional treatments are needed and call back this afternoon. States there has been remarkable improvement since first seen and he now gets around quite well. (Later): Client needs 20 treatments altogether.
April 2	Sent work letter.
April 5	Client returned work letter form: "I have not returned to work."
April 11	Client called and states that he has seen his doctor because of a foot condition and the doctor feels he needs special orthopedic shoes. Will call doctor regarding this. In general, he states he feels pretty good but his shoulders and hands are sore and stiff. Is still "too bunged up" to go back to work, but he wants to and will as soon as he is able.
April 15	Called internist regarding orthopedic shoes. Nurse states she will discuss this with him and have him forward prescription or have him recommend a podiatrist for an examination.
April 16	Doctor's nurse called. The doctor doesn't want to make out a prescription for orthopedic shoes but wants client referred to a podiatrist. He has no preference. If the podiatrist has any questions or problems, he should be instructed to call the internist.
April 17	Client chose a podiatrist. Letter and authorization sent to podiatrist for examination regarding orthopedic shoes.
April 23	Letter to client notifying him of authorization for four

office visits and X-rays for treatment of foot condition by the podiatrist.

April 25 — Report received from podiatrist done April 18 and April 23, recommending X-rays of feet and rubber molded appliances. The doctor states, "This patient in my opinion will be helped only slightly with any type of appliances as his systemic condition limits the effectiveness of this type of therapy." (Editor's note: The client later said the molded insert appliances changed the weight and pain to another part of the foot, so he took them out.)

April 26 — Called podiatrist who states padding helped some, but would like X-rays of both feet to determine if a light-weight brace would be appropriate. In cases of systemic arthritis a shoe, brace or any other weight often is more harmful than helpful. At any rate, his present shoes are adequate. X-rays and 3 or 4 office visits would help to determine what appliance, if any, is necessary. Will contact if authorization necessary. Appliance would be indicated for improvement in light of overall condition.

May 14 — Verification of increase in disability payment received. Form 0-300 previously submitted on Feb. 8. Send work letter.

May 20 — Work letter received. Client states, "Not employed."

May 24 — Received podiatrist report of five office visits: "The X-rays revealed severe arthritic changes in the tarsal region of both feet, also a marked osteoporosis due to the inactivity of the patient. Positive galvanic therapy did not help. Rubber molded appliances were placed in a suitable lightweight oxford and the patient reported that these seemed to help so that he could get around for about 3 to 4 hours without pain. Any improvement beyond this point will probably depend upon his general response to medication by his internist."

May 27 — Called client. He states his shoulders are still quite inflamed and he has been having enough trouble that he can't return to work yet. His internist has sent him to the physiatrist for instructions in home exercises and these have helped some. He doesn't think he will have to go to physical therapy any more.

May 29   Letter to internist asking for his comments regarding patient's present condition, the prognosis and the possibility of returning to work. Enclosed a copy of podiatrist's report.

May 29   Received physiatrist's report of examination on May 22: "Examination today reveals that the patient has been having considerable pain in both feet and he has been to a podiatrist. There is a fungus infection healing and he has had a soft insert prescribed for both feet. He was encouraged to continue walking even though there is a fair amount of pain in the feet; but not to overdo it. The knees reveal the previously noted edema on the left side with moderate instability of both knees; right greater than left. The shoulders reveal about 65-70 degrees of rotation, all of which is external rotation and the left shoulder has about 35 degrees of external rotation. Abduction is to 90 degrees bilaterally with the last 10-15 degrees being assistive. All of the ranges are within the functional range and he is totally independent in the activities of daily living. It is therefore necessary for him to continue these activities in order to maintain the existing range and he was encouraged regarding various exercises in order to maintain his present level of function."

June 19   Processed bill for hospital out-patient physical therapy, 25 treatments.

June 21   Letter received from internist: "Mr. David Willson has had a remarkable return of function. His arthritis is relatively quiescent. He is slow in his ambulation but he is able to get around with reasonable speed. I believe he is at maximum improvement at the present time and would be capable of working at a job not requiring

Rheumatoid Arthritis

undue physical exertion." (Editor's Note: client later said he felt his improvement was due to the overall therapy and bufferin.)

June 21   Called client. He wants to return to work, but still has pain in feet, legs and shoulders. Thinks he could do work where he would not be on feet too long. Would take company job at the factory. Has difficulty lifting nine pounds, but thinks he could do bench work. Has operated cash register when he worked in produce business, but no other business machines. Has been mixer, sweeper and guard at the factory.

June 27   Called on Mr. Grover High, factory personnel manager. He states that the client has been given progressively lighter work because of his disability for nearly 20 years, and at present there are no lighter jobs available because of automation. The client worked as a mixer for 12 years and then as a machinist, janitor and guard.

July 1   Mrs. Angle from the YWCA called to request a man to do light janitor work and operate an elevator, plus act as a security guard: hours from 5:30 to 11:30 p.m., salary $1.25 per hour. He could have a stool in the elevator. May have to set up extra card tables and empty some waste baskets, must be responsible. There is another applicant and she will call me within the next 2 days regarding the possibility of placement for this client.

July 8   Client called and was informed of job possibility at YWCA. Is interested. Also interviewed for job as ticket taker at theater but has not been hired as yet. Left word for Mrs. Angle to call. Mrs. Angle called and said to have client call for appointment for job interview. Youth Corps client originally had job but quit. Called client. He will make appointment today and inform me of results.

July 22   Called client. He talked to Mrs. Angle who stated she would consider him for something the first of September. At present she is involved with the Job Corps trainees and in the process or reorganization. He definitely would like to get this job which involves operating an elevator; however, he would take another position and is willing to work for $1.25 per hour. He had operated his own business at one time and feels that he could operate a cash register easily as he is good with change and figures and has been fairly fast with an adding machine. Will check with Mr. John Black and call client back.

July 23 Called the podiatrist and internist for billing. Will send billing in, pronto. Hospital reports client's last visit was March 28.

July 25 Called John Black. Is interested in client for possible cashier's job and will interview between 2 and 5 p.m. on Friday. Called client and will meet him at the restaurant about 5 p.m. July 26.

July 26 Met with client and Mr. Black regarding placement as a cashier at the restaurant. They will begin him on a four hour part-time schedule beginning July 27. He seemed to understand what was involved and no problems are anticipated. Mr. Black requests a clearance from his doctor on TB. Will call if any problems occur.

July 29 Letter to internist regarding TB clearance for job as restaurant cashier.

Aug. 1 Reviewed case. Will follow up on placement and request to internist next week.

Aug. 6 According to John Black, the client is doing very good work. He is going to take him on at $2.00 per hour as a cashier. Still wants a TB clearance. Called doctor's office to send TB report.

Aug. 9 Report received from internist: "Mr. David Willson is presently under my professional care. He is free of any communicable diseases including tuberculosis."

Aug. 12 Sent copy of doctor's report to Mr. John Black at the restaurant.

Aug. 20	Received progress report from internist: Mr. David Willson has continued under my medical supervision and has continued to do well. He receives 50 mgms of Solganol every 2 weeks in addition to taking salicylates. He is not on any cortisone or any other antiinflammatory drugs. He has some good days and some bad days but generally is reasonably pain free and comfortable. Most recently he has returned to a part-time job as a cashier in a restaurant and is seemingly adjusting well to this. I believe that we should continue Mr. Willson on the present schedule of gold therapy for an indefinite period of time. The dose, however, may be decreased in quantity or frequency depending on his symptoms."
Sept. 3	Talked to client on the phone. Will check after doctor's visit Sept. 19 and call us. Called doctor's office. Last office visit authorized was used Aug. 29. He is now on 3 week intervals at $9.00. Doctor will send invoice, and bill client for future visits. Case ready for closure after billing.
Sept. 5	Billing cleared on case.
Sept. 8	Employment letter inquiry form showed $80 weekly pay as restaurant cashier, effective July 27.
Sept. 18 Status 26 Closed Rehab	Closed case report and report to Social Security Administration.
Sept. 19	Letter to client notifying him of completion of services and closing records.

David worked in the restaurant part-time, two hours a day. He made $100 per month, plus his Social Security pension and the rent from a small house he owned. He could walk a little in the yard that summer, and his daughter took his wife to the store. David could drive, but drove very little because his feet were too tender to push the brake very hard. His boss said David was very reliable, courteous and honest. He was never late, although his boss knew he had a difficult time to make it some days because of the pain and stiffness. He had quit taking the gold shots when the agency quit paying for them.

He continued through the winter as a cashier until June of the following year when he went to Ohio on his two weeks' vacation. Mr. Black wanted him to come back, but expected to close the restaurant soon, so David didn't return to work. The restaurant closed in July.

David knew a friend who got tools through the rehabilitation office, so he thought he would try to get a machine to make metal Social Security cards and sell them. However, the agency said it wouldn't pay.

He waited on customers at a fruit and produce stand nearby, sorted fruit and did other display jobs where he could both sit and stand and work on the days he felt like it. He played rum for high stakes (he once won $138) at the Moose and neighborhood taverns, but didn't drink. He did get a job as a watchman, a security guard at an insurance company building. He checked the buildings and could sit down when he wanted to. He did have to climb some stairs and that hurt his feet, but he got through the winter, although every few weeks a pain in his groin would hit and then go away.

Finally, at 5 a.m., after walking the floor since 3 a.m., one April day, the pain was intolerable. He went to the hospital and was operated on for a growth on the colon. A few days post-operatively, during a coughing spell, the incision burst and he was rushed to the operating room. For six weeks he was semi-conscious, not knowing what was happening to him. He had two operations for an aneurysm of the abdominal artery, and an amputation of his left leg following gangrene, with a stump revision 10 days later, above the knee. Two weeks later, his right leg was ampuutated below the knee. He was discharged in September and came home, where he reads a little, watches TV; his children visit him, and his wife helps him with whatever he needs. He has a wheelchair and a Hoyer lift, and he gets up about noon. He can sit till his legs hurt and exercise his fingers to prevent the contractions from becoming worse. But the exercise of the fingers starts the legs to hurting after a time, so he stops that, and when his legs hurt too much, he goes back to bed, usually in the early evening. He refused public aid which he sought to pay the $3000 hospital bill above the $14,000 paid by insurance. He would have been required to sell his house that was bringing him some rental money each month, and he didn't want to do this. The years go by slowly since he left the hospital.

David Willson is not especially cheerful, but neither does he complain. He takes each day as it comes. He did not reapply for rehabilitation services, nor was he referred. He sees nothing that could have been done differently to prevent his present disability, although he felt a great need for a therapist to come to the home at only a nominal charge which most people could afford. Ten dollars a treatment was more than he could pay.

From the evidence on hand at closure, the client seemed to be in a satisfactory situation with an understanding employer at a reasonable wage and improved physical condition; however, in the end, the business failed, the employment was only 2 hours a day instead of full-time as reported, and the ebb and flow of arthritis symptoms continued to fluctuate, requiring indefinitely continuing, costly gold therapy. Although probably not able to work full-time, the client was not employed at his maximum physical, mental, social and psychological capacity.

There were conflicting reports of the length of time of onset of the arthritis, and in spite of the physiatrist's report early in the case that the onset of arthritic symptoms followed the loss of his son, there was no psychological evaluation to explore the possible effects of what could be severe emotional trauma. Neither was there a social worker's evaluation of the family and the degree of influence its nearby members may have had on the client and his plans, aims and efforts. The whole family is quite close, with the children and grandchildren often running in and out of the house to say hello and talk with the grandparents.

The counselor was necessarily concerned with the mechanisms of authorizations, reports and bills, and he made quite complete entries in the chronological record. He did a good deal of work in his placement efforts.

For this patient, the evaluation and treatment by the podiatrist had little or no effect on his improvement physically. Otherwise, he was under the care of American Board certified specialists. It is not likely that the abdominal operation and ensuing amputations could have been foreseen since the climax in an emergency hospital admission occurred 19 months after the case was closed. An agency policy of periodic followup, such as is done in services for the blind, would uncover the need for assistance at a time when it is most useful.

DISCUSSION QUESTIONS

1. Discuss the "arthritic personality": Does it exist? If so, what is it?
2. Discuss the side effects of analgesics and their vocational implications.
3. Discuss the vocational implications of rheumatoid arthritis.
4. Discuss gross-motor and fine-motor skills in relation to progressive rheumatoid arthritis.

SUGGESTED READING

Acker, M. Vocational rehabilitation of the rheumatoid arthritic. J Rehabil, 23:12, 1959.

Brown, R. and Lingg, C. Musculoskeletal complaints in industry, annual complaint rate and diagnosis, absenteeism and economic loss. Arthritis Rheum, 4:283-291, 1961.

Carek, R. Rehabilitation following surgery for chronic arthritis. Rehabil Counsel Bull, 5:212-214, 1962.

Chalmers, R.M. The general management of rheumatoid arthritis. The Practitioner, 208:5-9, 1972.

Clark, W.S. Arthritis and rheumatism. J Rehabil, 31:10-12, 1965.

Hardy, R.E. and Cull, J.G. Severe Disabilities: Social and Rehabilitation Approaches. Springfield, Thomas, 1974.

Hollander, J.L., (Ed.) Arthritis and allied conditions: A textbook on rheumatology. (7th ed.) Philadelphia, Lea & Febinger, 1966.

King, S.H. Psycho-social factors associated with rheumatoid arthritis, J Chronic Dis, 2:287-302, 1955.

Kirchman, M.M. The personality of the rheumatoid arthritic parient. Am J Occup Ther, 19:160-164, 1965.

Langi, V.F. Rehabilitation of the arthritic patient. Mod Treat, 5:1010-1012, 1968.

Lowman, E.W., (Ed.) Arthritis: General principles, physical medicine, and rehabilitation. Boston, Little, Brown and Company, 1959.

Lowman, E.W. Employability of rheumatoid arthritis: Emphasis of physical rehabilitation. Arch Environ Health, 4:502-504, 1962.

Mental problems in rheumatoid arthritis. Br Med J, 4:319, 1969.

Moos, R.H. Personality factors associated with rheumatoid arthritis: A review. J Chronic Dis, 17:41-55, 1969.

Moos, R.H., Solomon, G.F., and Lieberman, E. Psychological orientation in the treatment of rheumatoid arthritis. Am J Occup Ther, 19:153-159, 1965.

Polley, H.F., Swenson, W.M., and Steinhilber, R.M. Personality characteristics of patients with rheumatoid arthritis. Psychosomatics, 11:45-49, 1970.

Robinson, H., Kirk, R.F., and Frye, R.F. A psychological study of rheumatoid arthritics and selected controls. J Chronic Dis, 23:791-801, 1971.

Rusk, H.A. Rehabilitation medicine. (3rd ed.) St. Louis, The C.V. Mosby Company, 1971.

Scoth, N., and Geiger, H.J. The epidemiology of rheumatoid arthritis: A review with special attention to social factors. J Chronic Dis, 15: 1037-1066, 1962.

Seidenfeld, M.A. Arthritis and rheumatism. In J.F. Garrett and E.S. Levine (Eds) Psychological Practices with the Physically Disabled. New York, Columbia University Press, 1962.

Chapter 14

THE DRUG ABUSER

    Case Study One
    Case Study Two
    Case Study Three
    Case Study Four
    Case Study Five
    Discussion Questions
    Suggested Reading

CASE STUDY ONE

R. J. A.
Black Male 15
Single
Completed Ninth Grade
Mental Retardation (Full Scale I.Q. 76) and Drug Abuse

Referral Source:

    Mr. A. was referred by the adolescent clinic of a local hospital where he was being seen due to drug abuse. The doctors there found him not addicted to heroin, the drug he was experimenting with when sent, but felt that in a little more time he would have been addicted.

Social Data:

    Mr. A. is a fifteen-year-old Negro boy. He dropped out of school when he was fourteen. He states that he is not interested in school and had experienced behavioral problems. He is interested more in obtaining vocational training and finding permanent employment. Apparently he receives little guidance at home. His mother works as a teacher's aide; his father gives him little time. He lives in an area of the city where there is not much for him to do, but where drugs are readily available. Mr. A. is the sixth of seven children. The youngest child at home is fourteen.
    Mr. A. was close to his mother, according to her, until recently. His

mother's chief complaint now is that he explodes easily. She also complains that: things have been stolen from the home; he stays out all night; he has mood swings and is quite irritable; he also refuses to obey his parents and lives independently from other family members. Mr. A's mother suspected that he was on drugs. His mother describes him as a follower, but as having many friends. He looks up to only one family member, an older brother in the service.

Mr. A. began to have difficulty in the public schools when in the third grade. He was hostile and showed signs of aggressive behavior. He received psychological examinations three times while in school. It was finally the school psychologist who referred Mr. A. to the adolescent clinic.

Psychological:

Mr. A. has a history of psychological evaluations – one while he was in the fourth grade. He was performing at the second grade level. During testing he showed a lack of interest and attention. He became so engrossed in one particular aspect of a problem that he missed the correct solution.

The psychologist writes that Mr. A. is characterized by preoccupation with threatening aspects in the outside world. He feels that he has been so thoroughly mistreated by adults – most particularly his father – that he continually has to be on guard against attack. Mr. A. feels that the world is so hostile that he cannot live in it without protection. Adults have failed to provide this protection; therefore, Mr. A. tries to keep the threatening or hostile aspects of a situation out of his awareness. By denial he divorces the act from the emotion.

In the classroom the threats and pressures are overwhelming. Mr. A. therefore, arouses appropriate emotions of his teachers or parents to create havoc, which also serves the obvious purpose of revenge against adults who have failed him.

It was recommended that Mr. A. receive as much attention as he could receive in a classroom and a minimum of pressure, which would best be accomplished in a classroom for the mentally retarded-educable. At any time that his functioning level returned, he was to be placed in a regular academic program.

Adults working with Mr. A. should receive an objective appraisal of his situation. When Mr. A. *throws one of his tantrums* he should be removed from his fellow classmates. This should be done in a non-punitive fashion in order to break the cycle he is perpetuating.

A psychological evaluation a year later by the same school psychologist, when Mr. A. was at age eleven, found his intellectual functioning higher. There was considerable evidence for organically based distortion of perceptions. Mr. A. had an accident when two years old which resulted in convulsions almost to the point of death. The school psychologist recommended that Mr. A. be allowed to experience success in school in order to enhance his low self-concept.

Mr. A.'s most recent psychological evaluation showed him still mildly retarded at age fifteen. The Wechsler Intelligence Scale for Children (WISC) gives him a Verbal Scale I.Q. 79; Performance Scale I.Q. 78; and a Full Scale I.Q. 76. Mr. A. had an open attitude toward vocational areas.

Medical Evaluation:

Mr. A. always has been in excellent health except for normal childhood diseases. At age 2½ he accidentally received camphorated oil and almost died from seizures. This occurrence now may be related to his low frustration tolerance and irritability. Findings of the last physical are indicated below:

HEIGHT:	65"
WEIGHT:	116 pounds
VISION:	Left, 20/30 without glasses Right 20/20
EARS:	hearing o.k.; canals clear; drums good
NOSE:	o.k.
SKIN:	color: Negro - pigmentation: dark
HAIR:	normal
MOUTH & THROAT:	oral: hygiene good; gums: healthy; tonsils: large; thyroid: not enlarged
LYMPH GLANDS:	Cervical: o; Supraclavicular: o; Axillary: o; Inguinal: few
THORAX:	o.k.
LUNGS:	clear
SCARS OR MARKS:	o
GENERAL APPEARANCE:	thin, muscular
B.P.:	120/170
HEART:	RSR ♂ ⓜ —Fb/min
ABDOMEN:	soft — non-tender

GENITALIA:	stage development IV; hernia: o; Pilonidal sinus: o
NEUROLOGICAL:	gait: n; coordination: good; strength: good; balance: good
FEET:	normal
POSTURE:	normal
HABITS:	o
MASCULINITY OR FEMINITY:	Masculinity
PERSONALITY TRAITS:	restless
POSITIVE FINDINGS:	fifteen-year-old; Negro male, healthy who needs positive direction
LABORATORY PROCEDURES ORDERED:	complete blood count
TENTATIVE DIAGNOSIS:	(1) adolescent adjustment Rxn (2) minimum cerebral damage – L Parietal due to camphorated oil ingestion at 2½ years.

Brief Description of the Patient and His Problems:

Fifteen-year-old Negro male referred by vocational rehabilitation for medical evaluation. Patient is acting out at home, i.e. staying out some nights; is an intermittent bedwetter; *put out* of school in ninth grade for playing hookey too much; and had F in all subjects.

Vocational History:

This client has no vocational history. He has just recently undergone work evaluation at the center. Before he was accepted there it had to be proven that he was off drugs. This fact was substantiated by periodic visits to the hospital where checks were made, including a urinalysis. At the center Mr. A. received evaluation in electronic assembly, welding, upholstery, carpentry, mechanics stockroom clerk and reading. He was recommended only for electronic assembly, and even here with reservations. All evaluators indicated that Mr. A. needed personality changes and recommended work adjustment training before training in any area.

Mr. A. has now completed his work evaluation. He is anxious to return to the center and begin work adjustment until he can obtain training in electronic assembly.

Since his evaluation, Mr. A.'s attitude has become quite positive toward a training program. He is receiving much support from home to begin training. He sees the reality of his situation, is not employed and looks forward to admission to the rehabilitation center.

Educational Evaluation:

Mr. A.'s intelligence classification in school was *borderline-slow learner.* He displayed marked hostility toward peers and adults. He had frequent tantrums. The highest grade completed was the ninth. Until he dropped out he was receiving passable grades and sometimes B's and C's. He received, however, all F's during his last semester due to too frequent absences.

Summary:

Mr. A.'s past history attained goals (vocational evaluation) and future objectives have all been indicated. Mr. A.'s main problems in the past, and still to be resolved in the future, are his impulse control, emotional problems and disruptive tendencies. Accompanying these problems he does have a learning disability which generalizes to all areas of learning endeavors. His work evaluation, and his positive attitude, plus family support, do give hope for future successes.

CASE STUDY TWO

R. E. S.
White – Female-18
Single
College Student
Drug Misuse Characterized by Inability to Adjust Socially and Vocationally

Referral Source

Miss S. was referred to voccational rehabilitation by Dr. Wilson of the City Hospital Adolescent Clinic. Miss S. has had a long history of adjustment problems and has a severe drug problem. She is presently on 35 mg. of Methadone per day.

Social History:

Miss S. is an eighteen-year-old white female who has graduated from high school. She lives with her father, mother, sister and three brothers. Her father is employed as a mechanical engineer at Phillip Morris and her mother works at St. Mary's Hospital as a medication technician.

She is a very attractive adolescent who has been on and off heroin, LSD and marijuana since she was fourteen years old. At age sixteen she was a self-referral to Dr. Wilson's Adolescent Clinic with the chief complaint being overweight and dysmenorrhea. Upon evaluation, she was referred to a psychologist who found she had a severe drug problem. From medical and psychological results it was felt that while she was treated for her medical problems, she should also be referred to a psychiatric social worker.

The social worker saw Miss S. and her family once a week for the next two years. During this time, she went through several traumatic experiences. The first was a friend's suicide resulting from an overdose of LSD. Some weeks later, a girl friend's father tried to seduce her. These two factors plus her own identity problem created an adjustment reaction with severe depression. During this period of depression she began living with her boyfriend who was also a heavy user of drugs and who was increasingly turning her on to heroin. Also at this time the family involvement with her psychiatric social worker became strained due to a disagreement between the father and the social worker. The social worker then contacted Dr. Wilson to inform him of present events.

Finally, Miss S. was arrested on drug charges and placed in a detention home. From a conference with Dr. Wilson, the parents, lawyer and the rehabilitation counselor, it was felt she would benefit from vocational rehabilitation and a Methadone program with supportive therapy. Based on these facts, Miss S. was released from the detention home.

Miss S. started taking drugs because "she thought her peers were boring doing childish things and she found herself hanging out with older people who turned her on to speed and then other drugs."

The family situation is strained. Miss S. states that she gets along with her mother as long as they don't talk about emotionally charged subjects. She feels her mother does not know how to relate to many of the things that she was experiencing. She does not get along with her father and sixteen-year-old sister but has a good relationship with her three younger brothers. Her concern is that her parents are inconsistent with her younger brothers as they were with her. She worries about her sibling's reactions as they get older.

Psychological Evaluation:

On May 18, 1971, Miss S. was referred by Mr. Moore of the Department of Vocational Rehabilitation to Dr. Silvers for a psychological evaluation.

The client was seen by the psychologists as an attractive older adolescent who was candid and cooperative throughout both the interview and test. She readily answered most of the examiner's questions as long as they dealt with purely factual material. When questioned about emotionally charged material, she answered perfunctorily but one time cried, became very angry and would not further discuss the topic. When asked what being drug free meant to her, she was unable to address herself to his question, and at this point cried. She admitted that she could not guarantee that she would not go back on heroin.

Evaluative Procedures:

Wechsler Adult Intelligence Scale
Rorschach Techniques
Thematic Apperception Test
Bender Visual Motor Gestalt Test
Sentence Completion Test
Informal Projectives
Human Figure Drawings

Objective Results:

Verbal Scale I.Q. – 128
Performance Scale I.Q. – 125
Full Scale I.Q. – 128

Miss S. earned IQs on the WAIS which placed her in the superior range of intelligence. In the verbal area her highest score was on social comprehension and judgment. In the performance area her highest score was on the ability to construct familiar objects from their component parts. In the verbal area her lowest score was on the ability to do abstract reasoning. It was felt that the obtained results were both representative of her present level of functioning and optimal for her at this time. No signs of organic brain dysfunction were noted.

Miss S. saw herself as a very angry young woman who was relatively ineffectual in her ability to express her feelings constructively. She felt strongly that she was not allowed a place in her life to use her intellectual resources but instead found herself punished for being intelligent and assertive. At present, she saw no possibility for a change in this attitude among the people with whom she had contact and saw herself as returning to heroin as an escape from these perceived pressures. Her primary response at present was depression and being fatalistic about life.

In general, Miss S. was a very immature, dependent, anxious adolescent who felt very inadequate and insecure as a person. Her social relationships were marked by flightiness and difficulty in forming close give-and-take relationships. She feared close relationships with other people and put emotional distance between herself and all others by emotionally withdrawing from them and isolating all feelings which she might have for other people.

She wanted to live away from her parents' home as she saw herself as controlled in all that she did. At the same time, she had little idea of how to care for herself in a mature way and had little ability to form mature interpersonal relationships. Her feelings toward her father were conflictual as she saw him as punishing and at the same time as promising emotional support to her. She almost completely denied the existence of her mother and no emotional alliance with her mother could be seen from the present information.

Overtly, Miss S. was somewhat guarded, mildly negativistic, and highly manipulative. Covertly, her major defenses were fantasy, rationalization, some intellectualization and repression. When faced with some emotionally threatening situation she had the ability to intellectualize and isolate all the affective charge of the situation. At the same time, she occasionally chose to respond to situations in an entirely impulsive fashion without at all thinking about the consequences of her behavior.

In summary, Miss S. was an adolescent of superior intelligence who saw herself as inadequate and insecure as a person and presented herself as an anxious, very immature, dependent young woman. She apparently had resorted to drug abuse in an attempt to gain some feeling of her own identity. She felt that any attempt to be herself and to use her intelligence was met with consistant punishment. She feared close emotional relationships and was likely to act out impulsively without considering the consequences of her behavior. In terms of helping her develop a more positive self-image, it is possible that she might benefit from a residential therapeutic community experience.

Medical History:

A medical abstract received from City Hospital reported that Miss S. was overweight and at the age of ten began to experience dysmenorrhea. Services were provided by City Hospital in the form of medication, physical therapy, exercise schedules and guidance concerning food intake. By the time of referral to vocational rehabilitation, her weight and menstrual problems were under control. Miss S. has experienced two *bombers* while on LSD and this disturbed her emotionally. The only serious medical problem from drug abuse Miss Scott has experienced is bronchitis resulting from smoking a large amount of marijuana. She has had no history of abcess or hepititis due to drugs.

PHYSICAL EXAMINATION:	City Hospital
GENERAL APPEARANCE:	Pleasant
HEIGHT:	63″
WEIGHT:	137½ lb.
VISION:	without glasses OD — 20/200 OS — 20/200 OU — 20/200
SKIN:	Oily
	Eruptions, Acne mild
	Icterus — no Pallor — no Palms — dry
	Hair — dry
EARS:	Hearing — normal Canals — normal Drums — normal
EYES:	Pupils: Equal — normal React to light — normal
	Accommodation — normal
	Extraocular Movements — normal
	Conjuctivae — normal
	Exophthalmus — normal
	Fundi — normal
NOSE:	Obstruction — no Sinus Tenderness — no

MOUTH AND THROAT:	Oral hygiene – good
THORAX:	Normal
LUNGS:	Clear
B.P. (recumbent):	130/70
HEART:	Normal
ABDOMEN:	Normal
GENITALIA:	Normal
NEUROLOGICAL:	Normal
FEET:	Normal
POSTURE:	Normal
POSITIVE FINDING:	Mildly Overweight
LAB:	CBC
	VA
TENTATIVE DIAGNOSIS:	Obesity, mildly due to excessive intake.

Educational History:

Miss S. graduated from a local high school where her performance was in the B and C range. It was felt by the school that she could have done better if she had tried. Miss S. enjoyed school to some degree and was interested in art and English. Her other interests include psychadelic music, nature and arts and crafts. She doesn't like sports. If it is possible for her to go to college she would major either in the area dealing with work in the field of parks and recreation or in arts and crafts.

Vocational History:

Miss S.'s previous work experience is limited. She has had only one job which consisted of operating the concessions at a local theatre during the summer. She earned $1.25 per hour. She first stated interest in arts and crafts. She has since mentioned several other areas of interest. These include social work, teaching, occupational therapy and possibly some type of job with Virginia Parks and Recreation.

Eligibility:

Miss S.'s primary disability has been diagnosed as drug misuse characterized by inability to adjust socially and vocationally. She is eligible mentally, physically, and financially for services of Department of Vocational Rehabilitation (DVR). She is currently seeing Dr. Wilson at the Adolescent Clinic and he is optimistic about her rehabilitation. Dr. Wilson feels that with Methadone maintenance and supportive counseling, guidance and therapy, this client can become a contributing member of society. DVR and Mr. Moore are in complete agreement with Dr. Wilson. Psychological, intelligence and aptitude tests also indicate that she is a capable individual. She enjoys art and hopes to take art education in college so she can become an instructor. Since this objective was in keeping with the client's aptitudes, abilities, interests, educational background and previous experience, it was felt that DVR services were justified.

Services:

This client will continue to be seen and treated by Dr. Wilson of the Adolescent Clinic for extensive guidance, counseling and related followup services at no cost to DVR. Along with the Methadone Maintenance Program and tuition sponsorship for college, DVR will offer supportive followup services in order to insure satisfactory placement and rehabilitation services.

Cost and Plans For Financing:

Eligibility based on need. The following was authorized:
City Hospital Methadone Program: ninety days Methadone at $1.50 day ... $135.00
City University: nine hours tuition at $19/hour 171.00
City University Bookstore: Books and Supplies 35.00
To Miss S.: twelve weeks of food allowance at $20/week 240.00

ADDITIONAL SERVICES:
Psychologist: Thirty therapy sessions at $30/each 900.00

Summary and Followup:

Miss S. left her home environment as recommended by Dr. Wilson of the Adolescent Clinic, Dr. Silvers, Clinical Psychologist, and Mr. Moore her rehabilitation counselor to attend summer school, in preparation for the fall semester (This was authorized by DVR).

THE FOLLOWING IS A RECORD OF HER PERFORMANCE AT CITY COLLEGE:
Principles of Act – C
Nonloom Techniques – C
Composition and Literature – Incomplete

After summer school, Miss S. was seen for an interpretive interview of the psychological evaluation which was administered prior to entering school. She concurred with most of the findings of the evaluation. Several therapeutic alternatives were mentioned including a half-way house out-patient facility and out-patient psychotherapy with a professional.

She did not feel that she could cope with the stresses of a half-way house either on an in-patient or an out-patient basis. She also seemingly did not give much consideration to entering psychotherapy on an out-patient basis.

A month later, Miss S. was admitted to City Hospital due to extreme emotional problems. This plus her inability to cope with the stresses of life necessitated her to be hospitalized on the psychiatric ward at City Hospital. Her parents hospital insurance covers the hospital cost but not Dr. Silvers fees, who has been seeing her in therapy.

After fifteen sessions of individual psychotherapy, Miss S.'s progress was slow, due to her lack of trust. Although progress regarding the sources of her problems has been slow, she has begun to show some positive practical behaviors regarding her future life. These behaviors have taken the form of asking to be withdrawn from Methadone and permission to begin looking for a job.

It was felt that Miss S. needed to continue with her hospitalization and psychotherapy. Fifteen additional psychotherapy sessions were then authorized.

Miss S. has continued her courses of treatment on the psychiatric ward of the City Hospital and has made considerable progress. Her relationship with her therapist has developed to a point of trust, and she is beginning to work through some of her problems. Presently, she has been working on the practical aspect of relating to others and on her disposition upon leaving the hospital. She has recently been talking about getting a job at a drugstore and living with her grandmother or getting a room in a boarding house until she can find a more suitable job and living quarters. These thoughts appear to be quite realistic and are being supported.

After the second set of fifteen sessions which were authorized, Miss S.

is still in need of continued psychotherapy. It is apparent, at this point, that any psychotherapy endeavor with her will be of a relatively long-term nature; however, once she leaves the hosptial, the frequency of therapy sessions will be considerably less than while she is an in-patient. She is making significant progress and is an excellent candidate for continued support by the Department of Vocational Rehabilitation.

Therapy continued with Miss S. on an intensive basis until she was discharged and placed on an out-patient schedule. It was felt by Dr. Silvers that Miss S. had all the necessary tools to function outside of a sheltered environment. Her future was discussed and she said that she did not want to go back to school. She also stated that she has a continued craving for heroin. This is not unusual as many ex-heroin addicts have this symptom after detoxification.

Miss S. left for California for a vacation. She felt this would enable her to think out the best course for her future. Mr. Moore, her rehabilitation counselor, placed Miss S. in status 24, services interrupted.

CASE STUDY THREE

J. P. O.
White — Male — 20
Single
Completed Ninth Grade
Acute paranoid psychosis and inadequate disorder and drug abuse

Referral:

Mr. O., along with his parents, felt the need of his hospitalization due to a rapidly developing psychotic episode which took place on February 4, 1973. Mr. O. later that week presented himself to the Georgia Regional VA Office for hospitalization.

Diagnosis:

On February 6, 1973, this eighteen-year-old, single, white male was admitted to a VA hospital. He was admitted for treatment of LSD, *speed* and marijuana. He was, on admission, markedly frightened and suspicious, inadequate, immature and withdrawn and presented himself as hostile and negative in attitude. He was diagnosed by the examining psychiatrist as having acute paranoid psychosis due to drug intoxication and an inadequate personality disorder.

On February 9, 1971, Mr. O. went to a second staff meeting. It was felt by the staff that he would profit by a further period of observation and hospitalization on a long-term basis in order to see how this would effect his future use of drugs. His parents were contacted, and they convinced him that a longer stay in the hospital would be for his betterment.

Evaluation:

Mr. O. and his parents were interviewed by a social worker in order to obtain a complete social history. Mr. O. was their first child after two years of marriage. He had temper tantrums as a child and frequently passed out from crying so hard that he quit breathing. He was an average student in school but did not participate in sports much, had very few friends, and felt uncomfortable with girls. In 1970, at eighteen years of age, he dropped out of school after completing the ninth grade because he could not adjust to the high school situation and had been in constant trouble with his teachers. He then went to work as an inspector at a screw machine company in Atlanta which manufactures nuts and bolts but worked there only nine months before enlisting in the Army. He joined the Army thinking that Army life would be pleasant, but he was disappointed and frustrated. While stationed in Korea, he began taking LSD in order to relieve his depression. After his general discharge from the Army under honorable conditions, he continued using LSD and other drugs, such as *speed* and marijuana, because he felt it was difficult for him to adjust to civilian life. He has been on thirty LSD trips during the past two years but stopped taking drugs very recently. He has recently worked for Goodyear for a month but quit this job because he was going to be *laid off.* He is presently unemployed.

His family life at home had always seemed economically comfortable, but his parents never had an overabundance of money. His father worked regularly and seemed strongly committed to the value of work and the necessity for hard work in order to get anywhere in life. Mrs. O. seemed to be a very warm and supportive person who is greatly distressed over her son's use of drugs. Mr. and Mrs. O. knew nothing of their son's drug episodes until February 4, 1973.

On March 7, 1973, Mr. O. was evaluated through the services of physical medicine and rehabilitation. His symptoms seemed to be in remission so he was assigned to manual arts therapy in the printing shop. He also was sent from a closed to an open ward and was given approval for participation in individual psychotherapy. He expressed interest in wanting to find a job and getting married upon his release.

On April 9, 1973, his ward requested that he be given psychological testing and counseling. He was given the Wechsler Adult Intelligence Scale, the Bender Visual Motor Gestalt Test, projective drawings and the Rorschach, partially in order to assess possible organic impairment caused by his drug usage. His test behavior was cooperative, coherent and relevant, and he manifested some interest in and motivation to succeed on the task involved.

Test results showed no organic impairment, and he functioned in the normal range on the WAIS. While he seemed to have the potential for bright, normal functioning, there were indications that emotional and environmental factors had interfered with this developing adequately. He performs well on tasks that require nonverbal skills, but not on the more academic, verbal and interpersonal tasks.

His performance on the projective measures indicated that his schooling and his relationship with his father were likely sources of his emotional and intellectual difficulties. His father is seen as a strong masculine figure, who apparently thought little of his son, and at least unconsciously made that quite clear. Unable to deal with these conflicts as he entered adolescence, he took the easy way out and gained status and acceptance in a *flunking* group. It seems that his present use of denial strongly interferes with his inter- and intra-personal problem solving.

It has been noticed that over the past three weeks his condition seems to be gradually improved through the use of medication and supportive therapy.

Provision and Arrangement of Services:

Mr. O. expressed the desire to get a high school diploma. On June 7, 1973, he took his General Educational Development test here and passed it. He seems to have shown quite a bit of improvement in his condition. He got detoxicated and later regained his balance. His idea of references and persecutory delusions have dissipated, and he has responded well to individual and group psychotherapy and counseling sessions. He has been home on several passes and has apparently refrained from taking drugs while there. He seems now to realize that he can get along much better without the use of drugs.

The Counseling Psychology Department administered the Lee Thorpe Occupational Interest Inventory and the Minnesota Vocational Interest Inventory. He showed interest in the mechanical field and expressed satisfaction at the possibility of working in electronics, being a pressman or a stock clerk.

The counselor contacted his former employer at the screw machine company, and this employer wanted to have him return to work there as an inspector. This was the same type of job he had previously before joining the Army. The counselor also told them about the GI Bill, so that he could get training at a later date in order to become a steam fitter. Mr. O. agreed to seek supportive therapy and counseling at a local mental health clinic.

Placement and Followup:

Mr. O. was discharged in August, 1973, and sent to the Regional VA Office. He was given a supply of medication – Mellaril: 50 mg. *q.i.d.* A copy of his discharge summary was sent to the office for followup care in order to help him with his level of medication and his family relationship at home. He will be living at home with his parents and is supposed to resume working at this former place of employment.

CASE STUDY FOUR

S. J.
Black Male 21
Single
Completed Eighth Grade
Schizophrenic, Reaction Paranoid type and Drug Abuse

Identifying Data:

Private S. J. is a twenty-one-year-old, single, black male who was referred to a general military hospital on February 23, 1971, for psychiatric treatment and evaluation. Patient had been on active duty for three years and was air evacuated from Germany with a diagnosis of schizophrenic reaction, paranoid type, secondary to alleged ingestion of LSD. He was alleged to have been involved in a homicidal act while in Germany.

Social Background and History:

Patient was born in California. His mother is a registered nurse and his father is an auto mechanic. Patient's parents were separated while he was very young. His father was described as being very cruel and often resorted to physical abuse of the patient. Relationship between mother and patient has been very poor. Patient lived with his grandparents until age sixteen. They were very religious and frequently used quite harsh disciplinary procedures particularly over matters involving social difficulties. The patient made an unsuccessful attempt to reside with his mother; however, because of frequent arguments and emotional outbursts, he was forced to return to his grandparents. The patient has one sister, age twenty, and one brother, age seventeen, who was described as being very jealous of and was constantly lying about the patient.

Educational History:

S. J. dropped out of high school in the ninth grade because of poor grades and entered the Job Corps for about one year. At the age of eighteen, he enlisted in the Army.

Military History:

The patient enlisted in 1970. Basic training was completed in California and the patient spent five weeks in flight school. He later was transferred to Germany. S. J. was AWOL from his unit in Germany from July, 1972, until his hospitalization in Germany.

Pertinent History:

The patient is suspected of murdering a German Caucasian woman with whom he lived for several weeks (while AWOL from his unit). He claimed that he was looking for a woman who would love him when he met this girl who worked in a night club as a stripper. He admitted to being on several drugs at this time: *hash, speed,* LSD, etc. Patient claimed that he thought the woman had been influencing his mind, that she and a Dutch sailor in the neighborhood were trying to control him. On the night of the alleged murder, the patient acknowledged having fought with the victim. He began hitting her with an iron rod. She ran out into the street and he followed her. Following the incident the patient was apprehended by the German police and turned in to the MP's who brought him to the emergency room where a psychiatric evaluation was performed. The patient at this time displayed bizarre and hostile behavior toward the examiner.

During hospitalization in Germany, the patient underwent psychological testing which "revealed data consistent with an illness of a schizophrenic nature in one with a limited intelligence." A Sanity Board

Proceedings Meeting was held and two diagnoses were given: 1. Brain syndrome, acute, manifested by alleged homicidal act, depersonalization, concrete thinking, paranoid and somatic delusions, auditory hallucinations, flat and inappropriate affect due to alleged ingestion of LSD; 2. Schizophrenic reaction, paranoid type, manifested by depersonalization, concrete thinking, paranoid and somatic delusions, hallucinations, flat and inappropriate affect.

The Sanity Board concluded that patient was unable to distinguish right from wrong, was totally deprived of the ability to adhere to the right, that his mental condition was such that he would be unable to cooperate intelligently in his own defense.

4/18/73

The patient was admitted to a general military hospital for treatment and final disposition. He gave the following account of the incident in Germany while AWOL from his unit. He stated that he no longer liked his unit, that he felt harassed there. He wanted to be transferred but was not allowed to do so. He claimed that he had wandered about the city and was kept by women because they "liked me." He stated that he had come to know the victim about one to one-and-a-half months earlier. During this time, he felt that she could read his mind, control it and his actions and was attempting to turn him against the German people. He stated that he saw her as two different people – one-half of her body as his mother and one-half of her body as herself.

At another time he saw her as a witch. He felt that she practiced black magic and could make things disappear. He also related that he had one-half of his body turned into a cat, that he frequently saw other people's faces change spontaneously into that of a cat or tiger. He claimed both he and the girl frequently used drugs together and many of the incidents previously mentioned occurred during their use. On the night prior to admission to the German hospital, he claimed that he had been given drugs by another person who lived with his girlfriend on occasion. He stated that he felt overcome, that his body and mind were not his own. He stated that he struck this girl (the victim) with a silver pipe, and then feeling that he killed her, attempted to commit suicide by forcing a spoon down his throat. He was unsuccessful, however, and ran into the streets after which he was arrested by the German police.

Psychological Evaluation:

Tests administered: Wechsler Adult Intelligence Scale (WAIS),

Draw-A-Person (DAP), Bender Visual Motor Gestalt Test, Rorschach Evaluation: The patient was found to be functioning in the dull normal range of intelligence (WAIS full scale I.Q.: 86). A comparison of current functioning with the premorbid capacity indicates that there is no general deficit in intelligence. His verbal and motor skills are generally comparable (Verbal I.Q.: 87, dull normal; Performance I.Q.: 86, dull normal). His profile of individual skills is variable. He is below average in all areas, with the exception of verbal concept formation. This pattern is not indicative of organicity. Rather, it suggests a schizophrenic process, with paranoid ideation prominent. There is no evidence of perceptual motor impairment. The patient's performance on the Bender Visual Motor Gestalt, while demonstrating an obsessive-compulsive style, contra-indicated organicity.

4/18/73

Physical examination was within normal limits. Mental Status Examination: On initial interview, the patient was cooperative in his behavior and appeared nonhostile in that he spoke in a quiet monotone throughout the interview. He appeared guarded and suspicious at times. He answered all questions briefly and volunteered no information. Speech pattern and psychomotor activity were not grossly unusual. He expressed ideas of reference, ideas of influence, visual hallucination and somatic delusions. He was oriented to time, place and person. No auditory hallucinations were elicited.

Hospital Course:

The patient was placed in closed ward status throughout hospitalization. He was started on 400 mg. of Thorazine per day. Dosage was increased to 1200 mg. per day due to persistent delusional material. Dosage was later reduced to 900 mg. per day. The patient participated in ward routine by attending meetings but remained silent. During the latter part of hospitalization, he became more seclusive, not wishing to participate in any meetings or activities. A work-up for organic pathology was done. EEG was mildly abnormal which might have been due to the high percentage of EEG abnormalities in schizophrenia and due to high dosage of Thorazine. There was no evidence of organic central nervous system disease.

Diagnosis:

Schizophrenic reaction, paranoid type, acute, chronic, severe, manifested by loosened association, flattened and inappropriate affect, autistic preoccupations, somatic and visual hallucinations; once reported auditory hallucinations, ideas of reference, ideas of influence, alleged homicidal act, concrete thinking, seclusiveness, stress and rejection by a person significant to him. Predisposition: Marked schizoid personality adjustment, impairment for further military duty, marked impairment of social and industrial adaptability.

Recommendation:

The patient was referred for in-patient hospitalization in a Veterans Administration hospital. He is considered to be impaired to a severe degree due to persistent delusional thinking. He was considered to be potentially dangerous to others. It was decided that he is unfit for further military duty and was referred to the Physical Evaluation Board for consideration of separation from the service.

The Army Physical Evaluation Board found S. J. 100 percent disabled and recommended that he be placed on the temporary disability retired list of the U. S. Army.

7/16/73

The patient was referred to a Veterans Administration hospital from a general military hospital to determine his service-connected disability and for psychological testing and evaluation. On admission, the patient did not show overt signs of psychosis. His effect was somewhat sullen and flat but was not considered schizophrenic in nature. He was placed on 50 mg. of Thorazine per day. Medication was later decreased and all medication was discontinued on 9/8/73. The testing done at the VA hospital showed a significant psychopathic deviate score on the Minnesota Multiphasic Personality Inventory. The rest of the profile was very normal with the second high peak on manic activities. This suggests that if the patient had a schizophrenic breakdown, it is almost in complete remission at the present time.

Hospital Course:

During hospitalization at VA, the patient, while in open ward, indulged in unacceptable behavior by striking other patients on several occasions and by drinking. The patient physically abused two patients in his ward. On another occasion he molested a young woman, following her around constantly, attempting to place his hands on her person. His behavior around the ward suggested a psychopathic pattern.

The patient's unacceptable behavior in an open ward caused him to be placed in a locked ward without privileges. While in the closed ward, the patient also physically assaulted an elderly patient. S. J. sometimes denied many of these incidents. Throughout his hospitalization at VA, the patient did not show discernible evidence of schizophrenia or other psychosis. His behavior without medication was not different than that when he was on medication. Psychological evaluation fails to confirm the previous psychologist's impression of schizophrenia. The conclusion drawn from studies and observations at the VA hospital indicates disagreement with a diagnosis of schizophrenia. It is the opinion of those at the VA hospital that the previously observed behavior was due to drug effect rather than a manifestation of psychotic illness.

Conclusion:

It was concluded that the patient does not have a service-connected disability as previously indicated. The patient is regarded as having a personality disorder, anti-social type and military service was in no way a causative factor nor was it contributory to it. Patient was considered to be mentally competent in all regards.

Diagnosis:

1. Personality disorder, anti-social personality
2. Below average intelligence.
3. Drug addiction, by history and admission.
4. Drug induced psychotic reaction.

11/21/73

The patient was transferred back to a general hospital. He was returned to the Army jurisdiction for final disposition.

CASE STUDY FIVE

R. J. R.
Black — Male — 18
Single
College Student
Drug Misuse Characterized by Inability to Adjust Socially and Vocationally

Referral Source:

Mr. R. was referred to the Department of Vocational Rehabilitation by Dr. Davis of City Hospital, where he was seen in a drug treatment clinic. He is currently on a Methadone Program and is in the detoxication process. Due to his drug problem he has been unable to keep a steady job.

Social History:

Mr. R. is an eighteen-year-old, Negro male. He dresses in a neat, modest style and apparently has good hygiene. His family consists of his mother, who works as a clerk; his father, a waiter in New York; two sisters — fifteen and seventeen — living with his mother; and two brothers — one attending Howard University and the other living with his father in New York. Mrs. R. apparently knows of her son's addiction. Mr. R's addiction created some *hassels* between him and his mother. There is no known history of drugs in any of the other family members.

Mr. R. was a dealer for six months before he began experimenting with drugs. He averaged fifty dollars to sixty dollars per day selling on the street. He began snorting heroin one and one-half years ago "to see what everyone got so excited about." After a few months of using this method, Mr. R. began mainlining to obtain quicker results from heroin. During his addiction, Mr. R. supported a big financial and pharmacological habit by dealing and hustling. His stealing, robbing and purse snatching brought him thirty-five to seventy-five dollars per day. For one year, he used heroin every day. He stated that his supply was endless so he never went four hours between hits. On the streets, Mr. R. was what is termed a *good junkie.* He was good to other junkies when they needed a hit and they were good to him. Most of his friends were junkies. He presently hits twenty to twenty-five caps per day. Although he is a drug addict, he denies any serious use of drugs other than heroin. Mr. R. has never used LSD, *speed*, or Seconal.®

Mr. R. has never been arrested for drugs but has had a long standing history of petty thievery and minor skirmishes with police. He presents a picture of *always out for a fast buck.* The attitude of Mr. R. seems somewhat *standoffish.* He expresses a desire to kick and wants a job, i.e., *good life.* His past work experience indicated an inability to hold a job due to his drug habit.

Medical History:

Mr. R. stated that he has had a previous history of asthma and was seen in the city hospital adolescent clinic four year ago. He was treated with desensitization injections.

The present medical problem is drug addiction. Mr. R. has experienced some sickness with drugs; i.e. abdominal cramps, rhinorrhea, nausea and vomiting. He has had no previous history of abcess or hepatitis due to drugs. Mr. R's general medical examination was conducted at the City Drug Treatment Clinic.

The examining physician feels that it will be a "long, hard road" for Mr. R. It was also felt that if the client would become employed he could better handle his time while on the Methadone Program. Boredom and frustration have caused addicts who had once kicked to go back on drugs. Mr. R. has in the past weeks become bored and frustrated due to the lack of a job.

Physical Examination:

GENERAL APPEARANCE:	Cooperative, calm, neat
HEIGHT:	6' 2"
VISION:	OD – 20/200 OS – 20/200
SKIN:	Color – Brown Pigmentation – Freckles, Dry Eruptions, acne – none Icterus – negative Pallor – negative Palms – dry Vaccination Scar – negative Other Scars – negative
HAIR:	dry
EARS:	Hearing – good Canals – clear Drums – clear
EYES:	Pupils – equal React to light – Accommodation
NOSE:	Obstruction – negative
MOUTH & THROAT:	Oral Hygiene – poor Gums – fair
LYMPH GLANDS:	negative
THORAX:	negative
LUNGS:	clear Equal breath sounds
BLOOD PRESSURE:	90/74
HEART:	Regular Rhythm
ABDOMEN:	Soft
GENITALIA:	negative

NEUROLOGICAL:	negative
FEET:	negative
POSTURE:	good
HABITS:	Nail Biting – negative Tic – negative
	Speech – negative
MASCULINITY or FEMININITY:	Masculinity
PERSONAL TRAITS:	Confident

Systemic Review

Headache: *migraines*
Hearing: negative
Colds: yes
Hay Fever: yes
Asthma: desensitization

Chest Pain: negative	Palpitation – negative Dyspnea – neg.
Cough: negative	Wheezing – negative
Appetite: yes	Indigestion – negative
Abdominal Pain: yes	Nausea – yes
Dysuria: negative	Frequency – negative
Joint Pain: negative	Athletic Injuries – negative
Thumbsucking: negative	Bedwetting – negative
Sleep: negative	Dreams – no
Exercise: negative	Fatigue Easily – negative

Positive Findings (include patient's needs)

1. Mild Photophobia
2. Stated desire to *kick* habit

Tentative Diagnosis

1. History of asthma (took desensitization injections)
2. Heroin addicted (admitted)

Disposition, Present Recommendations

1. Lab work
2. Followup on asthma if needed
3. Urine dark (question hepatitus)

After Mr. R.'s physical examination, he was placed on 40 mg. of Methadone with a urine check three times a week. Two weeks later his dose of Methadone was cut to 30 mg. He was placed on a detoxification Methadone treatment.

Educational History:

Mr. R. graduated from the local high school two years ago in a general program of studies. His performance in high school was below average. As the client progressed from one grade to the next, there was a deterioration in grades achieved. By his senior year, Mr. R. had only one course grade better than a D; however, he did obtain an A in industrial arts. Also, between the eighth and twelfth grade, Mr. R.'s attendance decreased substantially. His tardiness increased significantly over the five years. Mr. R. was not involved in any extra-curricular activity during his high school career. He is presently interested in training that would involve using his hands. He is especially interested in wood working and industrial arts.

On the SCAT given in the eleventh grade Mr. R. ranked in the 13 to 37 percentile on Verbal, 41 to 68 percentile on Quantitative and 30 to 42 percentile total.

Mr. R. indicated that he liked school but felt that it "did little to train him for work."

Vocational History:

Mr. R. has had several jobs each lasting only a brief time. His first was with a local restaurant where he was a kitchen helper. He earned $1.85 per hour. This job lasted one month with Mr. R. quitting due to his drug habit. His second job was with a large local department store. Here he was a stock clerk and earned $1.95 per hour. He was fired after two months because he missed work due to drugs. Next, Mr. R. was employed with another local department store as a night janitor, earning $1.60 per hour. He was fired from this job after four months for the same reason, i.e. missing work due to his drug habit. His last job was a janitor for a local insurance company where he also did some clerical filing. This job lasted for a summer at the end of which he was fired again for the same reasons.

Mr. R. expressed a sincere desire to work. This desire was one of the major reasons for his going for treatment of his drug problem. He is tired of losing jobs because of drugs. He wants to contribute to society and

Drug Abuser

receive some of the benefits of work.

He is interested in industrial arts training. He likes to fix things and "loves to work with his hands." Mr. R. wanted to go into a job that he enjoys and feels that "this is one step toward being straight."

Psychological Data:

No psychological test data was obtained for this case. From Mr. R.'s high school records along with the doctor's and rehabilitation counselor's observations, it was felt that Mr. R. was relatively well-adjusted. He did become bored and frustrated during the initial Methadone Treatment Program due to idleness. He does need support and guidance in facilitating better use of his time.

Initial Services

Due to Mr. R.'s need for immediate job placement a more permanent vocational objective was planned after Mr. R. was temporarily employed. Several employers were contacted and Mr. R. was employed with Town Auto Parts as a stock clerk. He was paid $2.50 per hour. He still expressed an interest in wood working. He investigated the wood working courses at City Technical School and was interested in the cabinetmaking course. After this visit Mr. R. quit his job and dropped out of sight. Several attempts were made to contact him but all were fruitless. After almost two months, he showed up at the rehabilitation counselor's office. He stated he had gone back into the streets dealing and occasionally using heroin. About three weeks ago he decided that he didn't want this type of life and went back on the Methadone Program. He realized he had made a mistake and this time he was going to stay off heroin.

Mr. R. was then sent to Youth Opportunities and to City Hospital to inquire about a job. Later that day Mr. R. returned informing the rehabilitation counselor that he had secured a position in the transportation department at City Hospital. The idea of attending the City Technical School Cabinetmaking course was discussed. Rehabilitation would pay for the first session and if he kept his job, he could pay for the second semester.

A Rehabilitation Plan Was Written:

Mr. R. was certified eligible for rehabilitation services. His disability

APPENDIX

CASE STATUS CLASSIFICATIONS

00	Referral
02	Applicant
04	6 months Extended Evaluation
06	18 months Extended Evaluation
08	Closed from Referral
10	Plan Development
12	Plan Completion
14	Counseling and Guidance Only
16	Physical Restoration
18	Training
20	Ready for Employment
22	In Employment
24	Services Interrupted
26	Closed, Rehabilitated
28	Closed, Not Rehabilitated after services were initiated
30	Closed, Not Rehabilitated before services were initiated

INDEX

A

Abdominal artery, 196
Abel, T.A., 7, 19
Above-knee amputee, 126
Abram, Harry S.
Acciavatti, Richard E., 61
Acidity Urine Test, 112
Acker, J.E., 72
Acker, M., 198
ADC (Aid To Dependent Children), 83
Adjustment reaction, 205
Adler, Alfred, 5, 12, 19
Adlerians, 12, 14
Adolescent clinic, 200
Advisory committee, 26
Aid to Dependent Children, 113, 115
  benefits, 117
  payment, 116
Aid to the Blind, 93, 111
Aid to the Permanently and Totally Disabled, 39
Alcoholism, 152
Altschuler, K.Z., 157
American Foundation for the Blind, 118
American Foundation of Epilepsy, 25
American Heart Association, 68
Amputee, 158
Amputee clinic team, 130
Anderson, Miles H., 183
Anderson, W., 31
Aneurysm, 196
Angina pectoris, 65
Anginal pain, 68
Anti-poverty agency program, 51
Anti-social personality, 220
Arteriosclerotic, 64
Assistive Devices for the Motionally Handicapped, 41
Asthma, 221
Attitude Towards Disabled Persons Scale, 7

Audiogram, 109
Auditory hallucinations, 218
Aurally-handicapped class, 154
Autosomal dominant trait, 122

B

Babbidge, H.D., 156
Bagley, C., 31
Bakker, C.B., 72
Baller, W.R., 86
Barkemeyer, L.E., 31
Barker, R., 9, 19
Barrell, R., 72
Barrow, L., 31
Basic skill training, 92
Bauman, Mary K., 97
Baus, G.J., 31
Behavior modification, 23
Behavioral problem, 200
Bellak, L., 72
Bender Gestalt, 49
Bender Visual Motor Gestalt Test, 206, 214
Bennett, George, 47
Best, C.H., 103, 120
Best, H., 156
Bigman, S.K., 157
Birch, J.M., 157
Black lung disease, 34
Blakeslee, Berton, 183
Blind diabetic, 104
Blind mannerisms, 93
Block, J.R., 3, 20
Blood sugar test, 112
Blum, Richard H., 227
Body image
  theorists, 14
  theory, 4, 5, 6, 11, 16
Borderline-slow learner, 204
Braille, 106, 107, 116, 118
Brandaleone, H., 72

Bronchitis, 208
Bronchodilation, 50
Bronstein, L.H., 73
Brooks, Roy W., v
Browder, S., 31
Brown, R., 198

C

California Department of Rehabilitation, 145
California Mental Health Analysis, 89
Canadian crutches, 129
Cancer, 122
Cardiac disease, 68
Cardiac personality, 72
Cardiologist, 64, 68
Cardiovascular disease, 62, 64
Carek, R., 198
Carroll, Thomas, J., 97
Case statuses (see Appendix for complete description)
　00 (Referral) 126, 185
　02 (Applicant) 63, 127, 185
　10 (Plan Development) 64, 127, 187
　14 (Counseling and Guidance only) 64
　16 (Physical Restoration) 128, 187
　18 (Training) 69
　22 (In Employment) 70
　26 (Closed, Rehabilitated) 47, 59, 102, 124, 134, 168, 195, 227
Caveness, W.J., 31
Central nervous system disease, 218
Cerebral Palsy Foundation, 161
Chalmers, R.M., 198
Chamber of Commerce, 66
Chambers, W., 72
Charles, D.C., 86
Chicago Lighthouse for the Blind, 93, 94
Chronic bronchitis, 50, 60
Chronic obstructive pulmonary disease, 60
Clark, G.R., 86
Clark, W.S., 198
Cleveland, S.E., 6, 19, 72
Cofer, J.S., 86
Cognitive fatigue, 49
Cohen, Burton M., 61

Comprehensive evaluation center, 158
Comprehensive rehabilitation facility, 51
Concentration abilities, 49
Convulsive disorder, 22
Cook, W.L., 72
Coronary sclerosis, 65
Cor pulmonale, 50
Cortisone, 195
County health nurse, 33
Crammatte, A.B., 156
Crippled Children's Service, 34
Cull, John G., v, 31, 47, 61, 73, 86, 98, 103, 120, 136, 156, 198, 227
Cummings, J., 72
Cutler, S. James, 136

D

Davis, K., 7, 19
Dawis, R.V., 47, 98
Defries, A., 31
Delusional thinking, 219
Deming, W.E., 157
Department of Education, 76
Department of Public Welfare, 113, 115, 117
Department of Vocational Rehabilitation, 210
Desensitization injections, 22, 223
Deskins, A., 31
Detoxification, 211, 223
　process, 221
Developmental Disabilities Act, 25
DeWolf, A., 72
Diabetes, 99
Diabetes mellitus, 100, 113
Diabetic, 173
Diaphramatic breathing, 50
Digoxin, 50
DiMichael, S.G., 86
Dinger, J.C., 86
Disarticulation, 129
Diuretics, 50
Division of Vocational Rehabilitation, 48, 62, 126
　counselor, 51, 58
Dovenmuehle, R., 74
Drug abuse, 200
Drug intoxification, 212

Dudley, D.L., 72
Dunn, O.J., 74
Dyspnea, 36, 68

E

Edema, 192
Educational level, 51
EEG (Electroencephalogram), 218
Emotional problems, 78
Emotional trauma, 197
Emphysema, 50, 60
English, R. William, v., 3, 7, 10, 14, 18, 19
Environmental factors, 59
Epilepsy, 21
Epilepsy clinic, 27
Epilepsy Foundation of America, 22
Epileptic personality, 22
Epi-Hab Workshops, 25
Eye diagnosis, 113
Eye examination, 90

F

Fabing, D., 31
Felton, J.S., 47, 103, 120
Financial status, 56
Fisher, A., 31
Fisher, S., 6, 19
Fisher, S.H., 73
Food stamps, 158
Ford, A.B., 73
Foster, J.C., 31
Fox, H.M., 73
Frank, D.S., 31
Freedman, Arnold H., v
Freeman, L.W., 47
French, J.J., 47
Freud, Sigmund, 41
Freudians, 14
Friesen, Staley R., 137
Frost, A., 47
Frustration tolerance, 202
Frye, R.F., 199
Functional ability, 171
Functional vision, 106
Furth, Hans, 142, 156

G

Gait training, 129
Gallup, G.H., 31
Gardberg, M., 73
Garrett, J.F., 86
Garris, A.G., v
Gastaut, H., 31
GATB Test, 81
GED (General Educational Development Test), 214
Geiger, H.J., 199
Gelden, E.F., 73
Gelford, D., 73
Gestalt Psychology, 6
Ginsparg, S.L., 73
Glass, Ann, v
Glaucoma, 113, 115, 173
Gold shots, 186
Gold therapy, 195, 197
Goldin, G.J., 31
Goldwater, L.J., 73
Gonick, M., 9, 19
Gordon, G., 7, 8, 10, 19
Gorelick, J., 87
Gozali, Joan, 86
Gray, R.M., 73
Group discussion, 94
Group psychotherapy, 214
Group therapy, 94
Gruneberg, S., 31
Guerrant, J.J., 31

H

Habilitation, 145
Hagan, J., 73
Half-way house, 211
Hall, C.S., 15, 19
Handicapped telephone users, 40
Haptic Intelligence Test for Adult Blind, 89
Hard-of-hearing, 141
   children, 142
Hardy, Richard, E., v, 31, 47, 61, 73, 86, 98, 103, 120, 136, 156, 198, 227
Haselkorn, F., 72
Hash, 216

Healy, J.E., Jr., 136
Hearing handicapped persons, 138, 141, 143
Hearing loss, 142
Heart Association Evaluation Unit, 62, 65
Heath, M.J., 73
Heber, R., 87
Heise, H.W., 136
Hellerstein, H.K., 73
Hemipelvectomy, 175
  amputation, 125
  prosthesis, 127
Hepatitis, 208, 222
Heroin, 200, 250, 221, 223
Hertzman, M., 7, 20
Hollander, J.L., 198
Holleb, A.I., 137
Holmes, T.H., 72
Hornsten, T.R., 73
Howorth, M.B., 47
Hoyer lift, 196
Hurst, J.W., 73
Hyperventilation syndrome, 65

I

Individual psychology, 4, 5, 11, 16
Insulin, 99, 173
Intelligence Test, 76
Intermittent positive pressure breathing, 50
Internist, 187, 192

J

Jackson, R.N., 86
Jaros, R.M., 31
Job Corps, 216
Job knowledge tests, 144
Job seeking skills, 95
Job training, 51
Johnson, D.L., 72
Jones, J.W., 98
Jousse, A.T., 47
Junkies, 221

K

Kallman, F.J., 157

Kaplan, S., 73
Katz, L.N., 73
Kelly, William D., 137
Kennedy, John F., 85
King, S.H., 198
Kirchman, M.M., 198
Kirk, R.F., 199
Kivitz, M.S., 86
Kleck, R., 31
Klinger, Judith L., 183
Knudson, Alfred G., Jr., 137
Kohl, H.R., 157
Kohler, W., 6, 19
Kram, C., 32
Kronenberg, H.H., 157
Kuder Preference Record, 54

L

Langi, V.F., 198
Lebovits, B.A., 73
Letson, L.L., 31
Levenson, R.M., 72
Levine, E.S., 141, 157
Lewin, B.A., 47
Lewin, M.A., 103, 120
Lewis, H.B., 7, 20
Li, Frederick P., 137
Lieberman, E., 199
Life style, 171
Linde, L.M., 74
Lindesmith, Alfred R., 227
Lindzey, G., 15, 19
Lingg, C., 198
Linton, R., 7, 19
Liposarcoma, 124, 125, 176
Lipreads, 144
Livingston, S., 32
Lloyd, T.T., 157
Lofquist, L.H., 47, 98
Logue, R.B., 73
Lowman, E.W., 198
Lowman, Edward, 183
LSD, 205, 212, 213, 215, 216, 217, 221
Lunde, A.S., 157

M

Machover, K., 7, 20
MacKane, K.A., 157

Makowsky, B., 157
Manual dexterity, 53, 56, 82, 110
March of Dimes, 45
Margolin, K.L., 31
Margolis, D., 74
Marijuana, 205, 212, 213
Martin, C.J., 72
Maurer, David W., 227
Mayer, J., 137
Mayes, T.A., 157
Mayo Tumor Clinic, 215
McDaniel, J.W., 3, 5, 10, 14, 18, 19
McLaughlin, Parnell, v
Medical evaluation, 23, 203
Medical examination, 76
Medical therapy, 50
Meissner, P.B., 7, 20
Mellaril, 215
Mental health clinic, 215
Mental retardation, 75
Mentally retarded, 76
 educable, 201
Merrit, W.H., 31
Methadone, 205, 221, 224, 225
 maintenance program, 210
Miller, E.L., 86
Minneapolis Society for the Blind, 105, 107, 110
Minnesota Multiphasic Personality Inventory, 109, 219
Minnesota Paper Form Board, 55
Minnesota Rate of Manipulation, 89
Moos, R.H., 199
Mordkoff, A.M., 74
Morgan, Clayton, 98
Morris, W.H.M., 74
Motorized wheelchair, 177
Mozden, Peter J., 137
Mund, Seymour, v
Myklebust, H.R., 141, 157
Myocardial fibrosis, 65

N

Nasal catheter, 50
National Student Defense Loan, 101
Neeley, Aubrey, vi
Neo-psychoanalytic theory, 5
Nervous examination, 135
Neurological difficulties, 92

Neurology, 23
Newman, L., 157
Nixon, R.A., 86
Nolan, J.C., 74

O

Oberle, J.B., 7, 19
Occupational Interest Inventory, 55
Occupational therapy, 108, 209
Ophthalmologist, 112, 113
Organic brain dysfunction, 207
Organic pathology, 218
Orientation mobility, 108
Orthopedic appliance company, 44
Orthopedist, 172
Oskansky, S.S., 11, 19
Osteopath, 132
Ostfeld, A.M., 73
Otis Quick-Scoring Mental Ability Test, 54
Otological exams, 154
Out-patient facility, 211
Out-patient psychotherapy, 211

P

Palpitation, 68
Parallel bars, 129
Paranoid psychosis, 212
Parsons, O.A., 74
Parsons, Talcott, 7, 8, 10, 19
Pathology reports, 124
Patterson, C., 32
Paul, O., 73
Pennsylvania Bi-manual Work Sample, 80
Perceptual motor abilities, 49
Perceptual motor impairment, 218
Performance evaluation, 77, 82
Perkins, D.C., 47, 103, 120
Perry, S.L., 31
Personal adjustment, 91
Personality disorder, 212
Personality evaluation, 49
Personnel tests, 144
Petrie, J.G., 47
Phantom pain, 126, 180
Phantom sensation, 126
Phelps, W.R., 86

Physiatrist, 184, 192
Physical distress, 70
Physical examination, 90
Physical therapist, 129
Physical therapy, 126, 180, 186, 208
Physically disabled persons, 7
Podiatrist, 191, 197
Pohlmann, K.E., 74
Polley, H.F., 199
Pond, D.A., 31
Popper, J.M., 6, 20
Portable oxygen equipment, 50
Porter, R.W., 47
Premorbid personality, 59
Pressure sores, 44
Prevocational evaluation, 51
Prosthesis, 125, 126, 172, 177
Prosthetic devices, 158, 169
Psychiatric evaluation, 216
Psychiatric social worker, 205
Psychiatric ward, 211
Psychiatrist, 212
Psychoanalytic theory, 11, 21, 16
Psychological evaluation, 23, 50, 136, 206, 217
Psychological examination, 76, 201
Psychological report, 81
Psychological testing, 108, 214, 219
Psychoanalytic theory, 4, 14
Psychological adjustment, 11, 12
Psychologist, 49, 206
Psychology of deafness, 145
Psychology of disability, 10
Psychomotor activity, 218
Psychopathic deviate, 219
Psychotherapy, 6, 15
Psychotic episode, 212
Psychotic illness, 220
Pulmonary condition, 48
Pulmonary department, 58
Pulmonary function, 50

R

Rancho Los Amigos Workshop, 161
Ranier, J.D., 157
Rasof, B., 74
Rehabilitation counselor, 77
Rehabilitation evaluation center, 85
Rehabilitation plan, 163

Rehabilitation psychology, 3
Reinhart, A.M., 73
Reiser, M.F., 72
Residential therapeutic community, 208
Respirator, 45
Respiratory problems, 49
Retarded
  mildly, 75
  profoundly, 75
  severely, 75
Retro-lental fibroplasia, 90
Rheumatoid arthritis, 184, 185
Richard, T., 32
Rizzo, N.D., 73
Robinson, H., 199
Robinson, H.A., 7, 20
Role-playing sessions, 144
Role reciprocity, 8
Role set, 8
Role theory, 9, 11, 14, 16
Rorschach, 49
Rosen, M.A., 86
Rosenburg, Charlot, 47
Rusk, H.A., 137, 199
Russell, E., 31

S

Salicylates, 195
Sands, H., 32
Sanford, G., 73
Sarbin, T.R., 8, 20
Sarcamatous degeneration, 122
Schilder, Paul, 5, 20
Schizophrenic, 215
  process, 218
School psychologist, 201
Schmidt, R.P., 32
Scoliosis, 122
Scoth, N., 199
Seconal, 221
Seidenfeld, M.A., 199
Seizures, 21
Self-concept, 6
Sensori-neural hearing loss, 154
Severe pulmonary problems, 59
Severely disabled, 71
Shekelle, R.B., 73
Sheltered environment, 77
Sheltered workshop, 56, 64, 82, 85, 92, 95, 159, 188

Sign-language, 145, 146, 152, 154
Silverstein, A.B., 7, 20
Skateboard, 169
Skimkin, Michael B., 137
Small Business Administration, 66, 69
Social casework, 136
Social evaluation, 23
Social history, 35
Social motivation, 5
Social relationships, 207
Social role theory, 4, 7
Social Security Disability benefits, 48, 62, 66, 163
Social Security Trust Fund, 58
 counselor, 55
Social work, 209, 213
Social worker, 51, 197
Sociopathic personality, 152
Solomon, G.F., 199
Sparkman, D.R., 74
Special education classes, 76, 85
Special education programs, 143
Speech discrimination test, 154
Speed, 212, 213, 216, 221
Spinal cord injury, 33
SSDI (Social Security Disability Insurance), 176, 178
State Employment Service, 58, 62, 117
State mental institution, 152
Steinhilber, R.M., 199
Stevens, H., 87
Stigma, 4
 by association, 11
Stotsky, B.A., 31
Strong Vocational Test For Men, 109
Stuckless, E.R., 157
Sugar Urine Test, 112
Supportive counseling, 210
Supportive therapy, 205, 214, 215
Sweet, W., 74
Swenson, W.M., 199
Switzer, M.E., 157
Syden, M., 87

T

Talking Book Service, 88
Taylor, N.B., 103, 120
Temkin, O., 32

Thematic Apperception Test, 206
Therapeutic environmental manipulation, 15
Thorazin, 218, 219
Thornton, John, 74
Tilt table, 126
Tizard, B., 32
Tobias, J., 87
Tosberg, William A., 183
Trianda, H., 32

U

Unemployment compensation, 48
Urinalysis, 204

V

Verbal tests, 142
Vernon, M., 157
Verwoerdt, A., 74
Vieth, Clinton, vi
Visual clues, 154
Visual impairment, 107
Visually impaired, 88
Vocational Educational Program, 76
Vocational evaluation, 39, 77
Vocational goal, 166
Vocational history, 203
Vocational interests, 55
Vocational objectives, 39
Vocational planning, 23, 49, 88, 91, 105
Vocational Rehabilitation, 203, 205
Vocational Rehabilitation Act, 75
Vocational rehabilitation agencies, 99
Vocational Rehabilitation Amendments of 1943, 85
Vocational rehabilitation services, 58
Vocational rehabilitation training, 200
Vogel, Victor H., 227

W

WAIS (Wechsler Adult Intelligence Scale), 49, 68, 89, 206, 214, 217, 218
Wapner, S., 6, 7, 20
Ward, J.R., 73
Wargensteen, Owen H., 137

Weaver, N.K., 74
Webb, John H., vi
Weinstein, M.R., 31
Welfare caseworker, 35
Welfare department, 158
Welfare recipients, 84
Werner, H., 6, 20
Wheelchair, 196
White, J., 74
Whitehouse, F.A., 74
Wilder, B.J., 32
Williams, B.R., 157
WISC (Wechsler Intelligence Scale for Children), 202
Witkin, H.A., 7, 20
Work adjustment training, 159, 204
Work attitudes, 144
Work behavior patterns, 91
Work evaluation, 23, 203, 204
  unit, 51
Workshops, 23
Work-study, 85
  program, 76
Wright, B., 9, 10, 14, 18, 19, 20, 74, 103, 121

Y

Yoder, Norman M., 97
Young, J.H., 20
Youth Opportunities, 225
Yuker, H.E., 3, 20